D0915861

Concepts in Cancer Care

A Practical Explanation of Radiotherapy and Chemotherapy for Primary Care Physicians

Concepts in Cancer Care

A Practical Explanation of Radiotherapy and Chemotherapy for Primary Care Physicians

JAY SCOTT COOPER, M.D.
Assistant Professor in Radiology

DONALD J. PIZZARELLO, Ph.D.
Professor in Radiology

New York University Medical Center
New York, New York

 Lea & Febiger • 1980 • Philadelphia

Library of Congress Cataloging in Publication Data

Cooper, Jay Scott.
  Concepts in Cancer Care

  Includes index.
  1. Cancer. I. Pizzarello, Donald J., joint
author. II. Title. [DNLM: 1. Neoplasms—
Therapy. QZ266 C777n]
RC270.8.C68 1980   616.99′4   80-10334
ISBN 0-8121-0716-0

Published in Great Britain by Henry Kimpton Publishers, London

Printed in the United States of America

Print Number: 3 2 1

To our families,

in appreciation of their love and support

PREFACE

Great strides recently have been made in our ability to care for cancer victims. Earlier diagnosis and improved treatment methods have saved many who, even a few years ago, would have been lost. But, concomitant with this happy development, there have been several changes. Whereas once there would have been only a few possible means of treatment, now there are many. The primary care physician, who often makes the first tentative diagnosis of cancer, may be confronted with a number of alternate possibilities for referral, posing difficulty in advising which one will be best for his or her patient. During and following treatment there may be reactions and complications, and their care may become the responsibility of the primary care physician assisted by the nursing and house staff. In short, care and management of cancer victims often falls, at least in part, to people who do not practice oncology as their primary specialty.

In this book, which is not intended to be an exhaustive treatise or treatment manual, we discuss methods and mechanisms of various non-surgical cancer therapies and attempt to explain the biological basis of each. Practical questions which commonly arise are explored. How does age or sex affect the choice of therapy? What role has cell type, degree of differentiation or anatomic location in choosing a particular mode of therapy? What complications may occur and what reactions? When may cure be the goal and when palliation?

This book is not intended for the cancer specialist. Our aim is to provide a rationale for cancer care that will be of value to the non-oncologist in assisting in choosing routes of referral, in advising his or her patient about what is to come, in helping the patient understand the reactions of his or her body to treatment and in managing the complications with which he or she may have to live.

We have constructed our book in three sections. The first is intended as background and contains an overview of clinical aspects of cancer. Some readers may already have much of this information in their body of knowledge and may wish to read it primarily as review. Others, perhaps less familiar with the material, may read it as new or updated information. In any case, it is the base on which the rest of the book is built and repeated reference is made to the information throughout the latter sections.

Next, the second part integrates basic science and clinical practice. The level is more complex and presumes that the reader has mastered the previous section.

Finally, the hazards, potential and unavoidable, of non-surgical oncology are described and explained in an attempt to present an even-handed evaluation of the state of the art.

Because this book is not intended for experienced oncologists, we have avoided highly technical language, precise dose designations and exact descriptions of methods of treatment. Our approach strives to be a blend of the conceptual and the pragmatic. We have attempted, and hope to have succeeded, in fusing explanations of the biological concepts governing choices in non-surgical therapy with practical advice about their consequences.

New York, New York   Jay Scott Cooper
                                                 Donald J. Pizzarello

ACKNOWLEDGMENTS

We gratefully acknowledge the assistance of the following persons in preparation of this book.

For review and valuable criticism of the manuscript we sincerely thank:

> Dr. Joseph Newall,
> Dr. Hy Kozak,
> Dr. Thomas Borok,
> Dr. Roma Gumbs

For a thorough reading and correction of the manuscript we thank:

> Dr. Seymour Cooper
> Elizabeth Hellman

For patient typing and re-typing of the final manuscript we thank:

> Constance Carvell
> Elsa Kuhling
> Janice Wright

For invaluable aid in preparation of the illustrations we thank:

> Georgia Rave

J.S.C.
D.J.P.

CONTENTS

THE HAZARDS

THE GOAL

THE
BACKGROUND

1

FACTS AND
PHILOSOPHY

Cancers differ from normal tissues. They grow more-or-less autonomously, beyond host ability to control them. They spread into and destroy surrounding tissues. They detach fragments of themselves, which travel throughout the host's body, and in new locations, lodge and begin new cancers. They derange the host's metabolism and cause "wasting." Finally, if untreated, they kill their host and when they do, die as well. No normal tissue exhibits such bizarre behavior. No doubt about it. Cancers differ from normal tissues. But do they really?

From the viewpoint of non-surgical oncology, cancers are not unique at all. In fact, they are far more similar to, than different from, normal tissues. Researchers have sought characteristics that sharply distinguish tumors from their normal tissue counterparts, but such distinctions have not been found. From the viewpoint of non-surgical therapy, neoplasms and normal tissues are so alike that cancers cannot be treated without also potentially harming the host. What are cancers? What are these things which, viewed from one perspective, hardly could be more abnormal, yet, from another, are so similar to normal? Where do they come from? And, how can they be controlled?

Origins of Cancers. Sometimes it seems as if cancer has only relatively recently afflicted mankind and that it is a uniquely human scourge. For example, characters in 19th century novels and operas usually fell prey to consumption, madness and pneumonia; rarely did they succumb to cancer. Why is that? Why not an occasional cancer? Was consumption more romantic? Or was cancer not a problem with which audiences could identify? Not so many years ago, cancer seemingly was little known, and now, it appears to be everywhere. There must be few Americans alive today who do not know at least one person who has had the disease.

Yet, cancer is neither new nor uniquely human. Malignant growth may well be as old as life itself. Tumors have been described in nearly all forms of life in the animal kingdom and neoplastic growth is well known in plants. Among humans, cancer has been noted in mummies preserved from ancient Egypt, and no reason exists to suppose it began there. Whatever cancer is, its distribution includes nearly all life forms on this planet, and it is certainly not new.

One, therefore, wonders: What accounts for the recent public awareness and concern about cancer? Some possibilities come to mind. Possibly the incidence of cancer *actually* may be greater now than in the past, or the incidence may not be greater, but is *perceived* as greater. Perhaps a combination of factors is at work.

Cancer is a disease associated with aging. In former days, many diseases claimed people's lives, frequently before they could become old. In the United States, modern medicine has reduced the threat of death by tuberculosis, pneumonia and diphtheria and improved sanitation drastically has limited, if not eradicated, plagues such as cholera, typhoid and typhus. People now live longer and consequently may fall victim to cancer. Had they lived in the past, they might have died too young to develop the disease.

In addition, the incidence of certain cancers has changed, some increasing, others decreasing. Additional use of carcinogenic substances may account for the increased incidence of certain cancers, in particular, those arising in the lung. But others, like those of stomach or uterus, for unknown reasons, have decreased substantially. Overall, the American Cancer Society[1] reports that the incidence of cancer has declined slightly over the past 25 years.

If there is no real increase, why then is there a perceived increase? Possibly improved diagnostic methods uncover more cancers at earlier stages than in the past. That, combined with better therapeutic techniques, results in a greater number of persons being alive with the disease. More people may be aware they have the disease and there may be more survivors. This is not a *real* increase in incidence, but it may give rise to the *illusion* of increased incidence.

Secondly, for some reason, cancer is a disease that has been socially unacceptable. Only recently have victims begun to disclose their illness, and even now a residue of the older attitude persists. Consider, for example, the awe engendered when Mrs. Gerald Ford, wife of the then President of the United States, announced publicly that she had breast cancer. Many congratulated her on her *courage* at having made such a public statement and expressed the hope that her example would encourage others to overcome their inhibitions and seek help early. With more people talking freely about cancer, there may be a perceived rather than real increase in incidence.

In a sense, however, it makes little difference whether cancer incidence is increasing in fact or in appearance. Cancer is a dread disease which the public wants cured. It is high on the list of national priorities and, for that reason alone, is a medical problem of the first magnitude.

Cancer as an Evolutionary Phenomenon. Independent of current perceptions, malignant growth is not new and appears to have been associated with mankind for many years. From the viewpoint of non-surgical oncology there are important implications in this statement. One of the most significant is this: Because cancers exist today, and presumably have existed for millennia, they must be reasonably well adapted for life on this planet. A basic tenet of biology states that life forms not well adapted or "fit" to the environment eventually become extinct, as natural selection operates against them. Cancer seems in no danger of extinction—at least not as a result of natural selection.

But cancers are not separate forms of life in the usual sense. They are composed of cells presumably *derived from normal tissues* of the individual in whom they live. Somehow, something happens to the genetic material—or to the expression of the genetic material—of one or a few normal cells in an individual. Whatever happens changes these cells, giving them the potential for malignant growth. Such genetically changed cells no longer are *identical* to those of the individual they arose in, and it can be argued that such cells and their descendants constitute a different organism, although closely related to the host. In a sense, they are a derivative parasite, living in the flesh of, and supported entirely by, the host from which they arose. Yet the change that creates this parasite is a limited one. Cancer cells evidently retain the memory of the successful evolutionary adaptations of their parent tissues, so that they, like their parents, can deal with most of the forces that threaten to eradicate life. However differently cancers behave, in the matter of survival from things that threaten life, one should *expect* cancers to have much in common with normal tissues. Although the genetic change that transforms normal cells into malignant ones confers a behavior that sharply distinguishes them from normal tissue, if that change also increased their vulnerability to the forces of natural selection, cancers either would have become extinct already or would be on their way to extinction. Since this is not the case, one must conclude that cancers are *no more* vulnerable to life-threatening forces than are normal tissue and whatever means one selects to try to kill cancers, in all likelihood, will have a high probability of killing normal tissues, too. This is not to say, however, that *no* differences between cancers and normal tissues exist which can be exploited in non-surgical cancer therapy.

In any non-surgical cancer therapy, agents already in existence in the environment of living matter are directed against the cancer. For example, ionizing radiation effectively destroys certain cancers. Yet ionizing radiation is part of the environment and a life-threatening force to which life forms are well adapted. Agents that prevent cell division are effective cancer chemotherapy. But such agents, in the form, among others, of plant alkaloids, form part of the natural environment and are agents to which living matter is well adapted. Still other substances damage deoxyribonucleic acid (DNA) causing cell death. In the environment, agents that do this occur naturally. Examples include ultraviolet radiations and various peroxides. Yet living matter apparently has found means for avoiding death as a result of attacks on DNA. In non-surgical cancer therapies, cellular structures, mechanisms and processes are attacked which are already protected by evolutionary adaptations. Thus, for therapy to succeed, the attacks must exceed the *capacity* of the natural protective mechanisms. *More* radiation must be administered than living matter can deal with during the time period encompassed by therapy. *More* peroxides must be administered than can be detoxified by cellular mechanisms in a given time. *More* mitotic inhibitors must be delivered than can be disarmed in a given interval. While both normal and malignant tissue can deal more-or-less effectively with *natural* levels of life-threatening agents, they may not be equally capable of dealing with *excessive* quantities. Differences in capability may not be great and may vary among cancers and normal tissues, but some do exist. The problem facing non-surgical oncologists, both now and likely in the future, is that *exploitable* differences are likely to be small. But it is just such small differences that will have to be exploited to prolong useful life for patients. Non-surgical oncology probably always will involve a degree of compromise. Some normal cells will be killed or changed during therapy and the number of normal cells in the affected individual will decline. But some cancer cells will also be killed or changed during therapy, and if therapy is to succeed, the reduction in cancer cell number should eventually exceed the reduction in normal cell number.

At present, consistent reduction of the cancer cell number to zero is not possible, because to do so would reduce normal cell number below tolerance levels. However, as research continues, more and more small but exploitable differences in the way cancers and normal tissues cope with therapeutic agents probably will be uncovered, and as a result, non-surgical oncology probably will become correspondingly more complicated. The oncologist will need to become more of a tactician, planning more involved strategies aimed at destroying cancer, selecting from a larger choice of methods which, together or in sequence, will best prolong the life of the patient. And yet, it is likely that there always will be reactions and complications, because *whatever* the oncologist chooses to do, inevitably will produce some normal tissue damage, destruction and/or compromise of function. Paradoxically, these reactions and complications often do and likely will fall into the province of the non-oncologist to recognize, understand and treat.

Surgical methods of dealing with cancer probably will remain relatively less complex, at least in theory. In a sense, a surgical procedure is a conceptually simple, although at times extremely effective, method of cancer control. Reduced to its most elementary form, if a cancer can be removed, it cannot threaten a person's life. Often, however, total removal is impossible. Too much normal tissue may be involved; the cancer may have metastasized; the patient may be unable to tolerate surgery; the cosmetic result may be unacceptable. In some cases, current non-surgical methods already produce cure rates equivalent to those produced by surgery with less morbidity. If lives are to be saved and morbidity kept at a minimum, non-surgical means must at times be used and be used wisely.

The Causes of Cancer. The view that cancer is a derivative parasite already has been introduced, and it is safe to say that most people studying the problem believe that cancers result from changes in the genetic material of normal cells. Several reasons compel acceptance of this hypothesis. For example, cancers do not have a unique histology, but can almost always be related to normal tissues from which they presumably were derived. Liver cancers are composed of malignant liver cells, kidney cancers of malignant kidney cells, breast cancers of malignant breast cells, and so forth. In addition, cancers "breed true." Within given organisms, cancer cells produce cells like themselves.

Even when cancers metastasize to other parts of the body, they retain their histologic identity. Cancers in experimental animals can be transplanted from one animal to another and when this is done, the transplanted tumor is composed of cells descended from the transplanted cancer, not transformed host tissue. Finally, in highly inbred experimental animals, strains have been found in which certain cancers develop in nearly every one of its members. Various mouse strains exist in which the probability of development of leukemia, breast or brain cancer is effectively 100%. This strongly indicates that such animals bear a *genetic* predisposition to the disease, a liability on the part of their particular genotype to change and produce malignant growth.

These observations speak for a specific genetic constitution for cancers which is passed on to and inherited by descendant cancer cells. The clear relationship to a parent normal tissue combined with the strong evidence of a characteristic genetic constitution point to the conclusion that cancers are transformed cells of the host's own body. Their "memory" of what they used to be is demonstrated by their histologic characteristics (liver cancers are identifiable as liver), but their unique genetic constitution is exemplified by the fact that they give rise to "offspring" like themselves, offspring that inherit and exhibit the malignant characteristic, autonomous growth.

If it is true that cancers are transformed cells of the host's own body, how do they occur? It is often stated that the cause of cancer is unknown, and in a sense that is true. But the contrary is also true. So *many* agents cause cancer and so many more are discovered yearly, that there seems to be nothing but causes of cancer. The multitude of agents that cause cancers are too numerous to catalog here, but they fall into three general, although extremely different categories: chemical agents such as aromatic hydrocarbons and azo dyes, biological agents such as viruses and physical agents such as radiation. It appears that cancer induction is a *common biological response* to many disparate stimuli. The common property of these stimuli is that they elicit a response called "carcinogenesis."

Carcinogens are believed to exert their effects by producing genetic *mutations,* and some of the mutations they cause result in malignancy. Mutations arise when a mutagen (such as carcinogen) causes an injury in the cellular genetic material which subsequently is repaired erroneously. Improperly repaired genetic matter may not function properly and, if so, results either in *non-functioning* genes or in genes which *function differently* than they did before injury. The changed status of the gene, a mutation, is permanent and heritable. When the mutation results in a particular type of transformation, the cell acquires the potential for malignant growth. But a cell or even a group of cells with malignant potential is not necessarily cancer.

Cancers are aggregates of neoplastic cells which have achieved autonomy, growing without homeostatic restraint and beyond control of the host. The means by which autonomy occurs is not known, but it seems that *autonomous* growth of cells with malignant potential will not occur, unless they receive a stimulus for growth. Interestingly, the cancer growth promoting stimulus need not be a carcinogen. Any growth promoting substance apparently will do. For example, hormones or hyperplasia-causing agents like croton oil or urethane can serve this purpose. However, the response of normal cells and malignant cells to these agents differ. When subjected to growth promoting stimuli, both normal and malignant cells will divide and hyperplasia results. But when the promotion stimulus is removed, normal cells cease growing. Cancer cells do not. Having once received the stimulus to grow, they continue to grow and thereby give rise to a neoplasm, a new autonomous growth.

This is not to say that *every* cell in a cancer ceaselessly will grow and divide throughout the natural history of the disease. It means only that cancer growth is beyond host control and usually with little host restraint.

Inevitability of Cancer Induction. Because of the immense range of substances which can induce cancer, some naturally occurring, such as ionizing radiations and viruses, and some man made, such as various industrial products, it seems likely that for many years to come, cancer will afflict mankind. This will be particularly true if society continues to increase its reliance on technology. Industrial wastes frequently are carcinogenic and it is difficult to dispose of them in ways that prevent their coming into contact with people—sometimes many years later. There are examples: Chemical wastes buried for 20 years have recently surfaced in upstate New York; radioactive wastes have leaked from underground vats contaminating the earth around them; smoke from factories, which is a kind of waste product, pollutes the air.

In other cases, society chooses to expose itself to carcinogens, when these carcinogens are beneficial or essential for other reasons. Examples range from ionizing radiations to automobiles. Ionizing radiations have immense medical benefits in both therapy and diagnosis so that society profits from their use, in spite of their proven carcinogenicity.

With continued research and progress, doses of medical radiation may be reduced and the fraction of the population exposed may be lessened, but people will continue to be exposed, probably in great numbers, because optimal medical practice demands it. Similarly, automobile exhaust contains carcinogenic substances. While the amount or perhaps the types may be reduced or changed, it is quite unlikely they will be eliminated or that automobile use will cease.

While automobile exhaust fumes and medical radiations are carcinogens which much of the population recognizes, there are many others which are much less well known. To cite a few examples, security devices at airports involve radiation exposure, many automatic switches use microwaves, some smoke detectors rely on radiations, and not a few medicines are carcinogens. Some skin preparations contain coal tars, and the same can be said for various shampoos. Even the cherished family TV set emits some radiation. But even if all man-made carcinogens magically could be eliminated, naturally occurring carcinogens would remain. Ultraviolet radiations from the sun, background radiation from the earth's crust and outer space, and carcinogenic viruses—to name only a few—would still be with us. All of this suggests that continued cancer induction is virtually assured, far into the future.

Cancer Frequency. Geneticists believe that all cells of the body are equally liable to mutate. Since cancers are most likely the result of mutations, they should occur in all tissues of the body and with equal frequency. Observations partly confirm this. Physicians know that cancer of just about every anatomical site has been reported. On the other hand, some cancers are common while others are rare (Fig. 1–1). The frequency with which cancers occur seems to follow two rules. All else being equal, cancers occur most often in tissues which are active in cell division. Cancers are frequent in hemopoietic tissue, mucosal linings and glands. Probably this relates to the promotional stimulus needed to produce cancers. While the genes of all cells are believed equally liable to mutate and, consequently, all are equally liable to malignant transformation, not all cells are subject to the same impulse to reproduce. Mitotically active tissues are subject to growth promotion. The cells of many such tissues have rather short lives. Dying cells constantly need to be replaced and to accomplish this, remaining cells are subjected to mitotic stimuli. This is characteristic of hemopoietic tissue and of the linings of the gut and certain glands. Other tissues may come under the influence of growth stimulation only periodically as occurs in human breasts.

1979 ESTIMATES

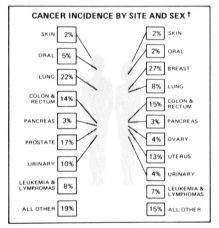

CANCER INCIDENCE BY SITE AND SEX †

SKIN 2%		2% SKIN
		2% ORAL
ORAL 5%		27% BREAST
LUNG 22%		8% LUNG
COLON & RECTUM 14%		15% COLON & RECTUM
PANCREAS 3%		3% PANCREAS
PROSTATE 17%		4% OVARY
		13% UTERUS
URINARY 10%		4% URINARY
LEUKEMIA & LYMPHOMAS 8%		7% LEUKEMIA & LYMPHOMAS
ALL OTHER 19%		15% ALL OTHER

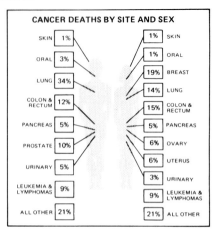

CANCER DEATHS BY SITE AND SEX

SKIN 1%		1% SKIN
ORAL 3%		1% ORAL
		19% BREAST
LUNG 34%		14% LUNG
COLON & RECTUM 12%		15% COLON & RECTUM
PANCREAS 5%		5% PANCREAS
PROSTATE 10%		6% OVARY
		6% UTERUS
URINARY 5%		3% URINARY
LEUKEMIA & LYMPHOMAS 9%		9% LEUKEMIA & LYMPHOMAS
ALL OTHER 21%		21% ALL OTHER

† Excluding non-melanoma skin cancer and carcinoma in situ of uterine cervix.

Fig. 1–1. *Cancer incidence and mortality by site and sex.* (1979 Cancer Facts and Figures. *Courtesy American Cancer Society.)*

However, this simplistic explanation must be incomplete because embryonic and fetal life, followed by childhood and adolescence are periods of intense mitotic activity but also are periods during which the frequency of cancer is *relatively* low. Why is this? Possibly, during intrauterine life, the filtering action of the placenta or of the mother's body protects the individual against many or even most carcinogens. Possibly, too, transformed cells are different enough from their host to be recognized as foreign and elicit a lethal immunologic response against themselves. The immunological system of an organism keeps surveillance over that organism, looking for objects which are foreign, ultimately destroying them. Perhaps in the case of recognition of transformed cells, immunologic surveillance usually is an efficient, but not *completely* effective, mechanism. Now and again the system overlooks or fails to respond to transformed cells. If this is the case, cancer should most often occur during periods of minimum immunologic competence—infancy and old age—and it does.

On the other hand, *for a cancer to appear,* it may be that mutant, transformed cells must undergo at least one more mutation, one which results in the loss of the antigenic markers that elicit immunologic response. Two *specific* mutations, occurring in the same cell would happen rarely indeed. Nevertheless, even though the probability is tiny, given enough time two specific mutations may occur in some cell somewhere in a body. If this two-mutation hypothesis is true, cancers would be expected to increase in frequency with advancing age—and they do.

No single hypothesis, however, fully explains the observed cancer incidence. Cancer is not a disease of the aged exclusively as the two-mutation hypothesis would predict. Cancer does not occur always when the immunologic mechanism is least efficient as the surveillance hypothesis would predict. Clearly, the picture is complex and probably all the elements are not known.

The second general rule of cancer distribution depends upon the concentration of carcinogens in the environment. If one marks the local frequency of occurrence of all cancers on a map of the United States, interesting patterns emerge. Certain regions have high frequencies of bladder cancer, others of lung cancer and so forth. Frequently these can be related—more or less tentatively—to ingestion, inhalation or contact with known carcinogens in the area.

Whatever the underlying explanations turn out to be, it is a fact that certain types of cancer are far more common than others.

Individuality of Cancer. Although various *types* of cancers certainly exist, every cancer is different from all others just as nearly every human being is unique. Since cancer cells are derived from cells of different individuals, they are as different from each other as individuals are from each other. Unfortunately, such subtle differences cannot be detected with the present state of knowledge, but they may be important determinants of the success of therapy. Consider, for example, treatment that depends upon minute differences between cancer cells and normal cells. Of necessity, the therapist usually will predicate his strategy on typical *average* differences between the cells. However, in a given individual, the difference may be significantly greater or less than this average, and the success of therapy can be diminished by as much as the individual varies from the average. Unfortunately, such individual variations cannot be measured *precisely* at present. Nevertheless, to the extent that it is possible to sense and compensate for deviations from the average, this should be done. With this in mind, the succeeding chapters discuss cancers and their management, both in terms of general principles for "average" lesions and moderating factors for the many nuances which may present in any case.

Reference

1. American Cancer Society: Cancer Facts and Figures 1979, New York, American Cancer Society, 1979.

2
BIOLOGIC
SPECTRUM

There can be little question that various types of cancers have inherently different personalities. Some appear content to grow by local invasion. Others metastasize widely, early in their course. And, one type may display varied behavior at different times depending upon its size or, by inference, the point at which it was diagnosed. In short, all cancers are not alike.

Logical assessment and management of a given cancer therefore requires an intimate knowledge of *its* particular biologic behavior. The site of origin, the histopathologic type, the signs and symptoms of disease, the mode of spread, the extent of disease, the options of therapy and prognosis, merely are the basic factors the oncologist must consider. However, as a first approximation, experience has shown that cancers which develop at the same anatomic site and have similar histology, tend to behave in a similar fashion. Thus, cancers can be grouped according to their site of origin.

The purpose of this chapter is to demonstrate the wide spectrum of personalities cancers display. To this end, a number of tumors, classified by site of origin, are presented. The selected tumors basically represent the major cancer sites as designated by the American Cancer Society: skin, lung, colon and rectum, breast, uterus and oral cavity. In addition, a limited sample of other sites has been appended; prostatic cancer—a common tumor with variable behavior; ovarian carcinoma—one fifth as common as uterine cancers but accounting for more deaths; and primary brain tumors—they do not metastasize, yet frequently are fatal. In sum, this chapter should serve not only to demonstrate the biologic spectrum of cancer, but also to introduce basic current concepts of management of several types of tumors, heavily weighted toward the common types the reader is likely to encounter.

Skin. Skin tumors account for the most common type of neoplasms. Fortunately, the usual histopathologic varieties also represent the most successfully treated tumors. Consequently, they are often overlooked in discussions of cancer.

Etiologically, these lesions often are associated with chronic irritants such as solar exposure. The common ones arise either in the basal or squamous cell layer of the epithelium of skin and as a result, basal cell carcinomas and squamous cell carcinomas account for nearly all such lesions.

Clinically, basal cell carcinomas classically present as translucent "pearly" nodules with elevated, rolled borders which contain minute telangiectatic blood vessels. Squamous cell carcinomas frequently have a superficially scaly or ulcerated appearance and bleed when manipulated, lacking the distinctive appearance of a basal cell carcinoma. But, both types of lesions take on many different appearances and it is sometimes impossible to differentiate between them clinically. Basal cell carcinomas nearly always occur on exposed areas, in particular the nose, eyelids and cheeks. Squamous carcinomas also tend to arise on the skin of the face but to a lesser degree; approximately one-fourth occur elsewhere. Both lesions grow almost entirely by local invasion and it is unusual for a cutaneous squamous cell carcinoma and rare for a basal cell carcinoma to give rise to metastases.

Because basal and squamous cell carcinomas tend to grow in a local fashion, many types of local therapy can provide successful management in most cases. For early lesions, surgical excision, surgical desiccation and curettage, radiotherapy or fresh tissue technique surgery (tumor is removed layer by layer for examination under the microscope, thereby permitting histologic guidance of the surgical procedure) produce eradication of disease in more than 95% of cases. Consequently, secondary factors such as cosmesis and simplicity can be used as the determinants of appropriate therapy. For large advanced lesions, where surgery would produce a significant cosmetic defect, for small lesions in delicate structures where surgery might produce a functional defect (such as an eyelid lesion), for lesions where the precise extension of disease is assumed to be substantial, but cannot be precisely delimited (for example, some lesions of the nose), radiotherapy offers a significant advantage over surgery. In contrast, when cosmetic changes are not important and when primary closure can be accomplished easily (as would occur with a moderate size lesion of the back) or in an area which will be subjected to considerable trauma (as occurs on the palms and soles), surgical management is preferable. Last, for recurrent lesions that have previously been treated inadequately by any method, fresh tissue technique surgery may permit more accurate exploration and therefore detection and treatment of tendrils of tumor trapped in the fibrosis caused by the previous procedure. If a patient acquires so many lesions that the previously discussed procedures would either not be possible or would lead to a mutilated appearance, topical chemotherapy in the form of 5-fluorouracil has been successfully used against basal cell carcinoma.[1] However, this form of management should not be used in the patient with only one or at most a few lesions.

Although relatively uncommon, malignant melanoma, should be mentioned because of its vastly different personality, when compared to the tumors just discussed. Malignant melanomas arise from pigment producing melanocytes, frequently within pre-existing benign nevi which are situated at the dermal-epidermal junction. Consequently, any change in the appearance of a pigmented nevus, such as an increase in size, alteration of color or bleeding should raise the suspicion of malignant transformation into melanoma.

Unlike the more common epithelial neoplasms of skin, melanoma behaves aggressively and frequently gives rise to lymph node and hematogenously borne distant metastases. To some extent the tumor's subsequent behavior can be predicted on the basis of its depth of penetration into subjacent tissue. Clark et al.[2] correlated decreasing survival with progressive invasion of deeper cutaneous layers. Similarly, Breslow[3] demonstrated that the depth of invasion (in millimeters) predicted the likelihood of metastases.

Clinically, melanomas acquire one of three appearances:[1] lentigo-maligna melanoma (occurs on exposed areas of elderly persons as a flat lesion of only slight invasiveness), superficial spreading melanoma (plaque-like lesions of variegated hues with some invasiveness in middle aged persons) and nodular melanoma (smooth surfaced spherical lesions of uniform blue-black color with primarily vertical growth into deeper tissues). As might be predicted, the prognosis of lentigo-maligna melanoma exceeds superficial spreading melanoma, both of which exceed nodular melanoma.

Treatment of localized malignant melanoma relies upon "wide and deep" surgical excision, including large margins of seemingly uninvolved normal tissue, with or without regional lymph node dissection.

(The value of node dissection in patients without clinical evidence of nodal disease, currently is subject to debate.) Lesions that have not spread to regional nodes can be cured in approximately 55% of cases; lesions that have given rise to microscopic size nodal metastases 30%; and lesions with clinically evident adenopathy about 10% of the time.[5] Symptomatic metastases can be treated either by radiotherapy[6] or chemotherapy[7] with the intention of producing palliation.

Lung. Carcinomas arising in the lung have recently become the second most common type of cancer to occur and, by far, account for the leading cause of cancer related deaths. In addition, the incidence of lung cancer has been increasing and continues to increase relentlessly every decade.

Carcinomas of the lung most frequently occur in the 50 to 60 year old age group and are associated with many kinds of irritants ranging from asbestos to tobacco smoke. Smoking 2 packs of cigarettes per day for 30 years results in a 1 in 20 chance of developing a cancer of the lung and a risk of death from lung cancer approximately 20 times greater than that of a nonsmoker.

Anatomically, nearly all lung cancers arise from the bronchi; three-quarters in a major bronchus and one-quarter in a peripheral bronchus. The lungs have a rich lymphatic network and tumors arising there have a propensity for lymphatic spread, draining into hilar, mediastinal and supraclavicular nodes. Axillary nodal involvement is not seen with localized lung tumors; the presence of axillary metastases implies involvement of the pulmonary pleura. As might be expected from its function in gas exchange, the lung also has a rich blood supply and metastases via hematogenous routes occur frequently.

Histologically most lung tumors are squamous cell carcinomas. Adenocarcinomas and undifferentiated carcinomas of both the large cell and small (oat) cell type are other frequently encountered histologies. Other histologic types are seen less commonly and, in terms of differential diagnosis, one must not overlook neoplasms which have metastasized to lung. Interestingly, the various histologic types display characteristic patterns of spatial distribution; squamous and small cell undifferentiated tumors most frequently arise centrally, near the mediastinum, while adenocarcinomas are usually considered peripheral tumors. All the common histologic types behave as aggressive tumors; however, small cell undifferentiated (oat cell) carcinomas have a particular propensity for distant metastasis. Eagan et al.[8] found that 47% of a series of oat cell carcinomas they studied had bone marrow metastases, and Newman and Hansen[9] found that 30% of their series gave rise to brain metastases.

Frequent symptoms include cough, which may produce increasing amounts of mucoid sputum, shortness of breath, pain and hemoptysis. Depending upon the precise location of the lesion, compression of the superior vena cava may occur (Chap. 12) or the lesion may invade various nerves. Involvement of the left recurrent laryngeal nerve produces hoarseness; involvement of the phrenic nerve produces elevation of the ipsilateral hemidiaphragm; involvement of the sympathetic system, Horner's syndrome of ocular meiosis, ptosis and ipsilateral facial anhydrosis; and involvement of the brachial plexus, severe pain in the arm and the shoulder. Some tumors also produce extrapulmonary manifestations (Chap. 15) including endocrine, neurologic, skeletal, dermatologic, hematologic and vascular changes.

Management of bronchogenic carcinomas, except for the small cell undifferentiated variety, employs surgery as the treatment of choice whenever possible. Morrison[10] randomly assigned cases to treatment either by surgery or radiotherapy. Six of 20 patients having surgically treated squamous carcinomas survived for 4 years, compared to 1 of 17 similar patients treated by radiotherapy. Unfortunately, only about one-half of all cases are suitable for operation and of these only half prove to be resectable at operation. When feasible, lobectomy is the procedure of choice.[11] It yields the same cure rate as pneumonectomy (with a lower morbidity rate), although for large lesions, pneumonectomy is sometimes required. Criteria for inoperability vary from surgeon to surgeon but the following provide a generally accepted list.[12]

1. Insufficient general condition to withstand surgery.
2. Extrathoracic disease or metastases in the opposite lung.
3. Small cell undifferentiated carcinoma.
4. Intrathoracic involvement of vital structures such as pulmonary artery or vena cava.
5. Vertebral or rib involvement.
6. Involvement of a major nerve.
7. Contralateral mediastinal nodal involvement or supraclavicular nodal involvement.
8. Pleural involvement, including malignant pleural effusion.
9. Tumor adjacent to or involving the tracheal carina.

Approximately 1 of 3 patients who undergoes resection is cured of disease. However, this reflects patient selection, the overall rate from bronchogenic carcinoma being between 5 and 10%.

For patients who refuse surgery or have an inoperable, yet *localized,* tumor, aggressive radiotherapy should be considered. Smart[13] produced a 22.5% 5-year survival rate by irradiation in a group of 40 technically resectable patients. Deeley,[14] Caldwell and Bagshaw[15] and Guttmann[16] each reported between 5% and 10% 5-year survival rates in large numbers of unresectable patients.

The primary limitation of radiotherapy in lung cancer does not result from an inability of radiotherapy to eradicate disease locally. For example, Bloedorn *et al.*[17] employed radiotherapy as a preoperative modality and were thereby able to compare the extent of disease found on histologic examination of the surgical specimen with the extent of disease, prior to irradiation. Moderate dose preoperative irradiation eliminated the primary tumor in 35% of cases and the mediastinal lymph nodes became negative in 77% of cases. Unfortunately these improvements in local status did not translate into improved survival. Failure of treatment in these patients, by implication, frequently must result from metastatic not local disease. In addition, these same authors[17] used preoperative irradiation to convert 36% of inoperable cases to operable ones. Unfortunately, this too did not improve overall survival. Other investigators usually have published similar results.[18,19] One notable exception occurs with apical pulmonary tumors. Such lesions appear to be less aggressive in terms of distant spread, and Paulson[20] was able to produce a 30% 5-year survival rate by the combination of preoperative radiotherapy and radical surgery.

The frequent appearance of metastases following local treatment of lung cancer has created a large population of patients that would benefit from effective systemic therapy. Unfortunately, such therapy has not been available. Traditional single agent chemotherapy, despite a large number of trials involving large numbers of patients who received a wide variety of drugs, has produced little if any benefit. Only recently have aggressive multidrug regimens begun to show some prospect of affecting the behavior of this disease. For example, Bitran *et al.*[21] produced at least partial tumor regression (Chap. 5) in 18 of 51 patients having metastatic non-oat cell carcinoma by administering a combination of cyclophosphamide, doxorubicin (adriamycin), methotrexate and procarbazine.

Because of the poor prognosis of patients who develop metastases, some investigators have electively administered chemotherapy to patients having *seemingly localized* disease in hopes of preventing the appearance of metastases. Such adjuvant therapy (Chap. 10), at most, has to eliminate only a small (clinically imperceptible) amount of tumor. Consequently, the drug(s) should be more effective than it would be against a large tumor burden. Unfortunately, thus far, such therapy has not been shown to improve survival.[19,22]

Oat cell carcinoma, in contrast, has a different response to therapy and requires no surgery other than biopsy for diagnosis. A randomized prospective trial by the British Medical Research Council[23] demonstrated that radiotherapy alone produced longer survival than did surgery in localized small cell undifferentiated carcinomas. Furthermore, oat cell carcinoma is relatively sensitive to available chemotherapeutic agents, which is fortunate in light of its high propensity for metastatic spread. The precise manner in which radiotherapy and/or chemotherapy will produce optimum management of this disease, however, has yet to be elucidated and several different regimens currently are being tested. For example, Choi and Carey[24] reviewed the course of 157 patients having small cell anaplastic carcinoma. Patients having initially "localized" disease fared equally well when treated by radiotherapy alone (reserving chemotherapy for progression of disease) or radiotherapy and elective chemotherapy either concomitantly or sequentially. In contrast, those patients having "extensive" tumors, experienced longer survivals after a combination of intensive chemotherapy and radiotherapy than after radiotherapy alone. Einhorn et al.[25] advocate adjuvant or therapeutic chemotherapy for all patients based upon improved survivals, compared to historic controls (Chap. 4), in their series. Both in their series and in the review article by Bunn et al.[26] elective whole-brain irradiation is recommended because of the substantial likelihood of cerebral metastases in this disease (Chap. 10). Unfortunately, average survival of patients having oat cell carcinoma after any form of treatment still is measured in months.

Colon and Rectum. Taken together, cancers of the colon and rectum occur approximately as frequently as cancer arising in the lung and account for the second highest annual death rate from cancer. Colorectal cancer affects both males and females with approximately equal incidence, two-thirds of the victims being more than 50 years old. Familial polyposis, ulcerative colitis, and villous adenomas predispose patients to this disease. Burkitt[27] suggests that the highly refined, low residue diets common in the United States, produce small quantities of infrequently evacuated stool which in turn permit various carcinogens to remain in contact with affected mucosal cells for long periods of time, and, therefore, account for the high incidence of this disease.

Histologically, these lesions tend to be well-differentiated

sidered, local recurrence was noted in over 90%, and it accounted for the *only* site of tumor in nearly 50%. Thus, the ability to decrease the incidence of local recurrence should provide great benefit.

Kligerman[41] has reviewed the results of pre- and postoperative combinations of irradiation and surgery for rectal cancers. The weight of evidence indicates that local recurrence is diminished, survival is improved and morbidity is no worse for the combined procedures than for surgery alone.

In contrast to the situation for radiotherapy, chemotherapy frequently is administered to patients having colorectal cancers, without substantial evidence of its value. Moertel[42] comments in this connection that "in many areas of this country it is only the rare patient who will escape some contact with 5-fluorouracil or the like at some stage of his disease." And yet, shrinkage of tumors by more than 50% of their size from these drugs occurs in only 15 to 20% of cases and such responses tend to be shortlived. Although some improvement in the response rate has been achieved by the combination of fluorouracil and a nitrosourea, no improvement in survival accrues.[43] Moertel[42] concludes that "chemotherapy of advanced colorectal cancer must remain an experimental endeavor."

In light of the disappointing results in advanced disease, attempts have been made to administer drugs earlier, before metastases have the opportunity to grow to detectable sizes. Despite numerous studies involving thousands of patients, prophylactic treatment has produced little to no improvement in survival. Higgins et al.[44] conclude that "there seems little reason to continue studies using 5-fluorouracil as a single agent." Currently, combinations of 5-fluorouracil and a nitrosourea are being investigated, but no firm data are available to attest to their efficacy.

The 5-year absolute survival figures nationwide[29] for colonic tumors demonstrate a 57% survival for localized lesions (approximately one-third of all cases), 36% for lesions with regional extension (approximately one-half of all cases) and less than 5% for lesions with distant spread (approximately one-sixth of all cases).

Breast. Breast cancer is the next most common malignancy and the most common cause of cancer related deaths in females. The disease has a wide variety of presentations, as well as behaviors. In some patients it proves to be rapidly fatal, while other patients manage to live in symbiosis with their disease for many years. In addition, the disease frequently proves to be hormonally sensitive and the clinical course and management in pre- versus postmenopausal patients, may differ significantly.

Breast cancer typically occurs in the perimenopausal period and appears to be related to an unopposed, prolonged estrogenic stimulus. For example, women who never were pregnant and therefore never had their menstrual cycle interrupted, have an increased incidence of breast cancer. Conversely, women who were pregnant before age 20 or who nursed their babies for prolonged periods or who had an oophorectomy at a young age appear to have a smaller risk of this disease.

The common mammary carcinoma arises from the epithelium of ducts within the breast and consequently is an adenocarcinoma. At first, the disease spreads through mammary lymphatics into axillary nodes, internal mammary nodes, and to a lesser extent, supraclavicular nodes. The likelihood and site of nodal metastasis depends upon size of the primary tumor and position of the lesion within the breast. Lane et al.[45] found that nearly 40% of lesions less than 1½ cm gave rise to nodal disease, while 70% of lesions greater than 4½ cm had such spread. Although lesions in the medial half of the breast are more likely to metastasize to internal mammary nodes than are lesions in the lateral half, axillary nodal involvement is more common than internal mammary involvement from any site within the breast. In fact, involvement of the axillary nodes (which are easily sampled) can be used to predict the likelihood of internal mammary disease. Patients with axillary nodal disease have an approximately 50% chance of having internal mammary involvement, whereas patients without spread to the axilla have a 20% chance or less of internal mammary involvement, depending upon the location of the primary lesion.[46]

Unfortunately, distant metastases from breast cancer occur frequently. To some degree, the likelihood of such metastases also can be predicted. Results of a national trial[47] reveal that patients treated by radical mastectomy who proved not to have axillary metastases, manifested distant disease within 5 years in only 19% of cases, while patients having 1 to 3 involved nodes experienced distant disease in 31% of cases. Those having more than 3 involved nodes suffered distant disease in 51% of cases. This amounts to a 76% 5-year disease-free survival rate in cases without nodal disease, a 48% rate in cases having 1 to 3 involved axillary nodes and an 18% rate when 4 or more nodes are involved.

Carcinoma of the breast usually is found as a painless mass within the breast, at times the tumor becoming attached to overlying skin causing dimpling or retraction of the nipple. One uncommon clinical variant occurs in the so-called inflammatory breast carcinoma which may result from a particularly aggressive tumor.[18] In such cases, the lesion rapidly occludes draining cutaneous lymphatics, causing a red, hot, swollen, tender breast which may appear inflammatory in nature. Biopsy frequently discloses plugging of dermal lymphatics by tumor. Patients having inflammatory breast carcinoma have an extremely poor prognosis and frequently die of metastatic disease within a short period.

Management of mammary carcinoma is both controversial and in flux. Disagreement about the preferred type of surgery, the roles of radiotherapy and chemotherapy all exist.

Traditionally, management of mammary carcinoma has required radical mastectomy, in which the breast, underlying pectoral muscles and axillary contents are removed *en bloc*. Not all lesions, however, are suitable candidates for this technique. In 1943, Haagensen and Stout[49] reviewed the clinical course of a large number of women who were treated by radical mastectomy and noted that certain characteristics of the tumor were associated with failure of the procedure. They codified these features into major and minor signs of inoperability; the presence of 1 major or 2 minor criteria indicating that the patient is not suitable for radical surgical management. In general, this concept has withstood the test of time, and the currently advocated criteria[50] are as follows.

Major Criteria
1. Extensive edema of the skin of the breast.
2. Satellite nodules in the skin of the breast.
3. Inflammatory carcinoma.
4. Parasternal tumor.
5. Supraclavicular metastases.
6. Edema of the arm.
7. Distant metastases.

Minor Criteria
1. Ulceration of the skin.
2. Edema of the skin of limited extent (less than one-third of the skin of the breast involved).
3. Solid fixation of the tumor to the chest wall.
4. Axillary lymph nodes measuring 2.5 cm, or more, in transverse diameter.
5. Fixation of axillary lymph nodes to skin or the deep structures of the axilla.

Five-year survival figures in breast cancer tell only part of the story. Because of the significant proportion of patients who display relatively slow clinical progression of disease, 5-year survivals for most forms of treatment are similar and only at 10 years or more are differences between various types of treatment evident. In addition, it is somewhat illogical to judge the efficacy of a local procedure, such as surgery, solely by overall survival rates when failure to cure so frequently is the result of metastatic disease. Consequently, for fair comparisons one must also look at local control rates in breast cancer. Prosnitz et al.[51] reviewed the literature and found that local recurrence rates ranged between 2 and 32% after radical mastectomy or variations of this procedure, extended radical or modified radical mastectomy. It is important to note that the time course for local failure is much more rapid than the time course of distant failure. Approximately 75% of local failures manifest within the first 3 years after surgery.[52]

In recent years, many surgeons have begun to use the modified radical mastectomy.[53] In this procedure, the pectoralis major muscle underlying the breast is preserved so that the contour of the axilla after surgery is normal in appearance. After appropriate case selection, the procedure is generally believed to be comparable to the classical radical; however, a prospective randomized trial to prove the modified radical equivalent to the standard radical has yet to be done.

Many years ago, McWhirter[54] suggested that simple mastectomy, preserving the pectoral muscles and the axillary contents, followed by postoperative irradiation to deal with any disease that may have been left behind by this less aggressive surgery, would produce similar results to radical mastectomy. Recently, the National Surgical Adjuvant Breast Project in the United States has conducted a randomized prospective trial of the necessity of radical mastectomy, randomizing patients between radical mastectomy and simple mastectomy followed by radiation therapy. The results of this trial[55] show no difference between the two forms of management.

Other physicians have taken this concept one step further. There are now several reports[51,56-59] indicating that local excision of small tumors followed by adequate irradiation of the remaining breast and draining nodal regions, produces survival and local control equivalent to more radical surgical procedures. Although the number of cases treated in this manner is not overwhelming and follow-up often is not extensive, a sufficient number of cases have been followed to permit preliminary analysis. The results of Harris et al.[59] are representative. Of 135 irradiated breasts, only 7 tumors (5%) recurred locally. Of these, technical factors accounted for some of the failures. None had received "booster" radioactive implants and 3 of the 7 occurred in patients who had less than excisional biopsy. In addition, cosmetic results were rated good to excellent by over 80% of sampled patients.

Thus far only local management of early breast cancer has been discussed. In 1975, Fisher et al.[60] reported on the use of L-phenylalanine mustard (L-PAM, melphalan) as an adjuvant to surgery to destroy occult distant disease and found a significant decrease in relapse rates for treated patients. In 1976, Bonadonna et al.[61] reported a similar trial using more aggressive and more effective chemotherapy consisting of cyclophosphamide, methotrexate, and 5-fluorouracil. Again, significant decrease in the relapse rate of treated patients was seen. Unfortunately, subsequent follow-up confirmed the activity of these drugs solely in premenopausal patients.[62] At 4 years 89.6% of premenopausal patients who received CMF were alive as compared to 70.6% of controls. The comparable numbers in postmenopausal patients were 76.5% in CMF patients vs. 75.4% in controls. Still, the concept of adjuvant chemotherapeutic management of breast cancer has been proven to be a realistic goal which currently is being actively pursued in many medical centers.

The role of radiotherapy as an adjuvant to surgery in "early" disease is controversial. For many years, in the United States, postoperative irradiation was administered to patients having primary surgical management of mammary cancer which had a substantial likelihood of failure to control disease at or near the site of resection. Although evidence to demonstrate improved survival resulting from the addition of radiotherapy is limited,[59] adequate irradiation virtually eliminates the chance of local recurrence.[52] However, recent availability of chemotherapeutic adjuvants to surgery has brought the necessity of adjuvant radiation into question. While a complete discussion of the many pros and cons of this argument is beyond the scope of this book, at least the following facts should be considered: (1) Adjuvant chemotherapy does not totally eliminate local recurrence. In the early report of Bonadonna et al.[61] 3 of the 11 initial recurrences in patients receiving CMF (compared to 7 of 43 initial recurrences in the control group) were completely within fields that could have been irradiated with conventional techniques. Although the numbers are too small to permit firm conclusions, the decrease from 7 to 3 local recurrences is not as good as would be expected from radiotherapeutic management. (2) If distant metastases are prevented from growing by chemotherapy, the relative importance of local recurrence increases. With CMF, local recurrences appear to be decreased only by the same proportion as distant recurrences. Thus, a method which could effectively eliminate local recurrences would have greater merit than in the situation wherein patients frequently die of distant metastases. (3) Adjuvant CMF chemotherapy does not appear to be effective in postmenopausal patients.[62] (4) Claims that radiotherapy of the chest wall produces significant clinical immunosuppression are unsubstantiated.[52,63] (5) Data from a randomized prospective trial testing the value of combining surgery, radiotherapy and chemotherapy are not available. Consequently, Harris' recommendations[59] that postoperative irradiation should be given to post-menopausal women who have either medial or central lesions and any number of positive axillary nodes or 4 or more positive nodes, and perhaps to high risk premenopausal patients would appear prudent at this stage of our knowledge.

Management of advanced, although clinically localized, breast cancer basically relies upon radiation therapy rather than radical surgery for local control. In general, doses which approach tissue tolerance are required, because of the volume of disease present and the well established relationship between volume of disease and dose required to control it (Chap. 10). After such treatment, local control of disease occurs in approximately two-thirds of patients.[64,65] On the other hand, occult metastatic disease frequently is present and adjuvant chemotherapy programs, as have been described previously, should be considered in such patients in the hope of improving the 5-year survival rates.

Management of metastatic breast cancer is reasonably successful. If all patients are considered, approximately one-third will respond to hormonal manipulation. The precise form depends upon the menopausal status of the patient and will be discussed in Chapter 6. In addition, chemotherapeutic management of disseminated breast cancer is also effective and this type of therapy will be described in Chapter 5.

Prostate. Following skin and lung cancer, carcinoma of the prostate is the most common cancer in men. After lung, colon and rectum it is the most common cause of cancer-related deaths in males. In addition, previously undetected microscopic foci of prostatic cancer not infrequently are found at postmortem examination, suggesting that the disease occurs even more commonly than it is diagnosed.

Classically, prostatic cancer has been described as arising in the posterior portion of the prostate gland, in contrast to the peri-urethral location commonly involved by benign prostatic hypertrophy. The overwhelming majority of such lesions are adenocarcinomas, most resembling to a considerable degree the normal prostatic cells from which they arose.

Initially, tumor grows by local extension, eventually penetrating the prostatic capsule and invading the seminal vesicles. Posterior extension, however, occurs only rarely; the tough fascia of Denonvillier protects the rectum from direct invasion. Early in its development, tumor also spreads by both lymphatic and hematogenous routes. Internal iliac and external iliac lymph node chains most commonly are involved, and, as might be expected, the incidence of lymphatic involvement increases with increasing size of the primary lesion. Palpable lesions confined to the prostate give rise to lymphatic metastases in up to 25% of cases, while tumors that have extended beyond the prostatic capsule involve lymph nodes approximately 50% of the time.[66] Hematogenous metastases secondary to prostatic cancer are common, in part due to access of tumor cells to the adjacent vertebral venous plexus of Batson. Bones, in particular within the pelvis, and the lumbar spine, are favored sites for metastases, producing relatively dense osteoblastic lesions.

Clinically, prostatic carcinomas produce few symptoms until they are advanced. Consequently, approximately one-half of all cases are diagnosed only after hematogenous metastases have developed.[66] An additional 5% of cases are diagnosed by accident when histopathologic examination of specimens obtained as part of treatment for benign prostatic hypertrophy are found to contain prostatic adenocarcinoma. In fact, the only reliable sign of *early* prostatic carcinoma appears to be distortion of the normal prostatic architecture by the tumor, which can be detected by examination *per rectum*.[67] Although elevated levels of serum acid phosphatase can be found in advanced disease, one would hope to detect lesions at an earlier stage of their development.

Not all prostatic carcinomas require treatment. Lesions discovered by accident, which closely resemble their parent normal tissue and which are found only in one small fragment of the resected specimen, are not likely to become a clinical problem during the lifetime of the patient and, in essence, require no treatment.[68]

Surgical management of prostatic cancers applies only to relatively early lesions, which account for only 10% of all prostatic tumors. Radical prostatectomy including removal of the seminal vesicles usually is recommended, and, as a consequence, 90% of patients who previously were potent become impotent and 15% develop urinary incontinence. Disease-free survival after surgery for lesions confined to the prostate varies among various reported series depending upon selection criteria but approximates 50 to 60% at 10 years.[69]

Radiation therapy of early disease offers an alternative to surgical treatment. The same volume as would be resected by prostatectomy must be irradiated and as a consequence approximately 25% of patients become impotent and approximately 5% sustain rectal damage. Survival is nearly identical to that obtained in the surgical series.[70-73]

For more advanced disease extending outside the prostatic capsule and beyond the limits of surgical resection, radiation therapy remains effective. Five-year survivals approximating 50% and 10-year survivals of 30% result after such management.[70-73]

Once disease has become disseminated, cure is no longer possible. If necessary, symptomatic relief should be achieved by the least aggressive means which adequately serves the purpose. If widespread symptomatic metastases exist, hormonal manipulation, either in the form of orchiectomy or administration of estrogens (Chap. 6), can produce palliation. In general, these procedures remain effective for 2 to 3 years. Subsequently other systemic measures including the administration of cytotoxic chemotherapy or radioactive phosphorus, both of which have some value, can be considered.

Cervix. Cancer of the uterus has two distinct forms depending upon the precise site of origin within the uterus. Carcinoma of the cervix occurs more commonly; however, in recent years the relative proportion of lesions arising in the cervix as compared to the uterine endometrium has decreased.

Carcinoma of the cervix typically affects the perimenopausal woman. It is more common in females who have a history of intercourse with numerous non-circumsized male partners and in females who began to engage in intercourse at an early age. Squamous cell carcinomas account for approximately 95% of all tumors arising in the cervix and the majority are moderately well-differentiated lesions. The posterior lip of the cervix is the most common site of origin and both exophytic and infiltrative types of lesions are common. Through routine check-ups and the use of the Papanicolaou smear, most cases of carcinoma of the cervix can be detected before they invade surrounding tissues or produce symptoms. When symptoms are present, they generally are related to changes in menstrual cycle such as menorrhagia or metrorrhagia. In postmenopausal women unexpected vaginal bleeding, especially after intercourse, is a common sign. A watery, yellow vaginal discharge may also herald carcinoma of the cervix.

Carcinoma of the cervix basically grows by local extension and invasion into the tissues lateral to the cervix. Extension anteriorly or posteriorly occurs less commonly. In addition, disease often spreads to regional lymphatics, the external and internal iliac nodes most frequently involved. Even if disease clinically appears to be confined to the cervix, approximately 15% of patients also have pelvic lymph node spread.[75] When disease has extended into the parametria, approximately 30% of patients have pelvic lymph node invasion, and, when disease has reached the bony sidewalls of the pelvis, approximately half of all patients have involved pelvic lymph nodes. With advanced disease, direct extension into the parametria can compress the ureters and thereby cause hydronephrosis. With advanced disease, direct invasion of the bladder, or, more rarely, direct invasion of the rectum can occur. Distant metastases are unusual, but when they occur, they generally involve either lung or liver.

Throughout the world, radiotherapy is commonly used for primary treatment of carcinoma of the cervix. Depending upon the precise extent of disease, the exact manner in which radiotherapy is given, varies. Frequently a combination of means is used—external beam irradiation to treat the entire pelvis, including the draining lymphatics, plus irradiation from a radioactive isotope placed within the uterine cavity and vagina (intracavitary therapy), to deliver a high dose to the volume affected by primary neoplasm. For carcinoma of the cervix, 5-year survival adequately measures cure. With modern radiotherapy, 5-year survivals approximating 80 to 90% can be expected when primary disease is confined to the cervix, and 60 to 70% when the disease has begun to penetrate the parametria.[76,77] Unfortunately, by the time the disease has extended to the bony pelvic sidewalls, only about 1 in 3 patients can be cured, and when disease is still more extensive, few patients survive 5 years.

Surgical management provides an alternative to radiotherapy in earlier stages of disease.[78,79] For disease confined to cervix or approaching the parametria, radical hysterectomy and pelvic lymph node dissection produces survival equivalent to that achieved by radiotherapy. Surgery, however, does require the patient to be in better general condition than is necessary for radiotherapy. In addition, if disease has invaded the parametria, surgery is not applicable. Radiotherapy, in such circumstances, offers the only hope for cure.

If the patient develops metastases, several different chemotherapeutic drugs including methotrexate, bleomycin and hexamethyl-melamine may produce transient remissions in approximately 25% of cases.[80,81]

Endometrium. Carcinoma arising in the endometrial lining of the uterus occurs in postmenopausal patients primarily. Approximately 90% of these tumors are adenocarcinomas, the vast majority being well-differentiated in nature. Such tumors are associated with prolonged estrogenic stimulation and victims also tend to be affected by obesity, hypertension and diabetes.

Clinically, most lesions are detected because of associated vaginal bleeding in postmenopausal women which ranges in nature from mild spotting to frank hemorrhage. Tumors arising in the uterine endometrium initially grow centripetally towards the uterine cavity, remaining confined to the uterus in most instances. To some degree they also grow centrifugally through the uterine myometrium and involve the uterine lymphatics and/or blood vessels. In the past, the frequency with which lymph node metastases occur, was not appreciated fully. Morrow et al.[82] present data gathered from the literature which indicate that lymph node spread occurs frequently in patients with invasive or poorly-differentiated lesions (Chap. 6). Although infrequent, distant metastases can occur. The lungs primarily are affected, most often with poorly-differentiated lesions.

Because endometrial carcinoma tends to present while clinically confined to the uterine cavity, surgical removal by total abdominal hysterectomy and bilateral salpingo-oophorectomy provides the basic form of management. However, in certain situations this procedure has shortcomings. When nodal disease is present, the operation obviously does not deal with such spread. In addition, approximately 10% of patients who have hysterectomy alone, subsequently experience recurrence at the upper vaginal vault. Consequently, some form of radiation sometimes is used in conjunction with the surgical procedure. When the primary lesion is well-differentiated and there is little or no invasion of the myometrial wall, there is little risk of pelvic lymph node spread. In such cases, hysterectomy alone may be sufficient; however, adjuvant irradiation decreases the chance of vaginal vault recurrence to only 2%.[82,83] On the other hand, for poorly-differentiated lesions or lesions which have invaded deeply into the myometrial wall, radiation therapy encompassing draining lymph nodes is advised. For lesions that appear poorly-differentiated on initial biopsy, some authors recommend that radiation be given preoperatively.[84,85] Once the tumor has reached the uterine cervix, initial management by radiation, followed in 4 to 6 weeks by extrafascial hysterectomy is recommended.[86] When extra-uterine pelvic structures are involved, definitive radiotherapy is indicated, with or without surgery, depending upon the clinical situation.[87]

For patients who are in poor general condition (and, therefore, are poor surgical risks), or have advanced lesions which are not amenable to surgical resection, radiation therapy alone should be used as primary management.[88] In such cases, treatment usually consists of both internal and external radiotherapy, although for early cases intrauterine therapy alone may suffice. While the degree of differentiation and degree of myometrial penetration in a given case influence the survival rate, overall, using treatment as outlined above, patients having lesions confined to the endometrium, have a 75 to 90% chance of 5-year survival.[89,90] Once the lesion has involved the cervix, 5-year survival decreases to 50 to 80%,[86,89,90] and, if pelvic structures also are involved, 5-year survival ranges from 25 to 60%.[87,89,90] If the lesion has metastasized, 5-year survivals approximate 10%.[89,90] For such disease, hormonal therapy in the form of a progestational agent produces remission in approximately one-third of cases (Chap. 6). Remissions may last for several years, particularly with well-differentiated, slowly growing lesions.

Ovary. Carcinoma arising in the ovary is the third most common female genital malignancy and is the number one cause of gynecologic-tumor related deaths. Most of these lesions occur in females between ages 40 and 60 and must be distinguished from the more common benign tumors of the ovary.

Ovarian carcinomas usually arise from cells of the surface epithelium of the ovary. They display a variety of histologies, the more common ones being serous cystadenocarcinomas, mucinous cystadenocarcinomas, endometroid carcinomas and undifferentiated carcinomas. In addition, a large number of uncommon histologic types of tumors occur, such as dysgerminomas, teratomas and granulosa-cell tumors.

Clinically, most ovarian carcinomas are diagnosed in an advanced state because of difficulties in detecting this disease. Abdominal bloating and lower abdominal pain are the most common signs and symptoms. Frequently, patients note that their clothes have become tight.

As a part of local growth, ovarian carcinomas shed metastases into the peritoneal cavity. This unique mode of dissemination creates a substantial problem of management. In addition, lymph node metastases and metastases apparently preferentially attracted to the medial aspect of the diaphragm have been demonstrated in a substantial proportion of patients.[91]

Optimal management of epithelial ovarian tumors is an unsettled issue. Surgery is considered the initial standard approach,[92] and whenever possible, total abdominal hysterectomy and bilateral salpingo-oophorectomy—with or without removal of the omentum—should be done. When disease cannot be excised completely, most experts advise removal of as much tumor as possible.[92]

The precise role of radiotherapy in management of ovarian carcinoma is subject to debate. In patients in whom gross lesions were confined to the ovary or ovaries, with or without malignant ascites, Hilaris and Clark[93] improved survival by instilling radioactive phosphorus into the peritoneal cavity and presumably sterilizing the remaining small tumor burden. When gross disease extends to the pelvis, it is generally accepted that surgery alone is inadequate therapy. Tobias and Griffiths,[92] in a review of the literature, demonstrated increased survival associated with subsequent radiotherapy. In such cases, even though disease appears to be confined to the pelvis, radiotherapy should be delivered to the entire abdominal cavity, as well as pelvis.[94]

Once disease has spread to the abdominal cavity, the ability to deliver cancericidal, radiotherapeutic doses is compromised by tolerance of surrounding normal tissues. Consequently, chemotherapy has been used with increasing frequency in such cases. Although it appears that any alkylating agent is effective, melphalan provides the common standard against which other agents or combinations usually are measured. Response can be expected in approximately 30 to 45% of treated patients,[95,96] and chemotherapy appears to be the best form of management when massive abdominal disease cannot be surgically removed. However, it is difficult to escape the conclusion that the precise roles of chemotherapy and radiotherapy in treatment of advanced ovarian carcinoma remain to be clarified.

Consider the following three series, each of which describes treatment of patients having advanced but less than massive abdominal disease. Smith and Rutledge[97] randomized patients to receive either radiotherapy or chemotherapy and found no difference between these methods. Buchler et al.[98] similarly found no difference between these methods, but noted that their data suggested improvement in survival when the modalities were combined. Bush et al.[99] reported a randomized trial which showed that abdominal irradiation plus pelvic irradiation was more effective than chemotherapy plus pelvic irradiation in controlling abdominal disease. However, a potential benefit of combining abdominal and pelvic irradiation with chemotherapy was also suggested, because they found improved control of pelvic disease in the group receiving pelvic irradiation plus chemotherapy.

Unfortunately, meaningful review of the literature is hampered by the recent appreciation of the frequency of nodal metastases. Previous radiotherapeutic programs may well have underdosed these regions. As a result, several new techniques have been developed, the methods of Fuks and Bagshaw[100] and Flink et al.[101] being representative. At the same time, new chemotherapeutic regimens are being studied. Although several attempts in the past at combination chemotherapy demonstrated no advantage over more conventional single agent alkylating therapy, Young et al.[102] recently reported improvement in survival of patients treated with a 4-drug combination; cyclophosphamide, methotrexate, 5-fluorouracil and hexamethylmelamine.

While these new programs offer hope for improved survival in the future, at present, 5-year survivals in patients who have lesions confined to the ovaries approximates 60%; for lesions extending to the pelvis 40%; and for lesions which have extended to the abdomen less than 10%.[92]

Head and Neck. Tumors which arise in the nasopharynx, oral cavity, oropharynx, larynx, and hypopharynx commonly are grouped together as head and neck cancers. More accurately, they should be separated into a larger number of categories, depending upon precise site of origin, such as cancers of the oral tongue, pharyngeal tongue, tonsil, aryepiglottic folds, vocal cords, and so forth. Tumors at each of these sites display their own unique personalities; however, to some degree, their similarities permit them to be discussed together.

Head and neck cancers disproportionately affect elderly males. Most victims frequently consume alcohol and use tobacco excessively. People of Chinese birth are prone to be affected by nasopharyngeal cancers. In the past, patients often had a history of syphilis; however, this is now uncommon. Approximately 90% of head and neck cancers are squamous cell carcinomas. The degree of differentiation varies with precise site of origin; tumors arising in the oral cavity tending to be better differentiated than more postero-inferior placed lesions in the pharynx. Unfortunately, patients who have a head and neck tumor are prone to develop a second independent primary tumor elsewhere,[103] particularly in the upper aero-digestive tract.

Clinically, cancers arising at each specific site within the head and neck region tend to be associated with specific symptoms. For example, carcinomas arising on the vocal cords characteristically produce hoarseness; carcinomas in the pyriform sinuses of the hypopharynx produce difficulty in swallowing; carcinomas of buccal mucosa can produce blood-tinged saliva; carcinomas of the nasopharynx can produce nasal obstruction or epistaxis, and so forth. However, some symptoms are common to several different sites (e.g., pain, either local or referred to the ear). While these symptoms usually force the patient to seek medical advice, at times primary lesions are clinically silent and lymph node metastases can be the first sign of disease, particularly with tumors of the nasopharynx, tonsil or base of tongue.

Both the precise site and frequency of lymph node metastases are characteristic of the specific site of origin of tumor. Upper jugular lymph nodes near the angle of the mandible are the most commonly involved site from all types of head and neck cancers. However, involvement of lymph nodes situated at the tip of the mastoid process (upper posterior cervical nodes) is suggestive of nasopharyngeal carcinoma, involvement of submandibular nodes suggests carcinoma of the anterior two-thirds of the tongue or floor of mouth, and retropharyngeal nodes (which may extend completely up to the base of the skull) are characteristic of hypopharyngeal cancers. Lindberg[104] has described the likelihood and position of clinical adenopathy present on admission in patients having various primary tumors of the head and neck. The rate of such spread is considerable from all sites but varies substantially: floor of mouth, 31%; oral tongue, 35%; soft palate, 44%; retromolar trigone and anterior faucial pillar, 45%; supraglottic larynx, 55%; oropharynx, 59%; hypopharynx, 75%; tonsil, 76%; pharyngeal tongue, 78% and nasopharynx, 87%. And even when clinical evidence of nodal disease is absent, subclinical disease frequently is present. Furthermore, the incidence of contralateral nodal involvement from lesions of the tonsillar fossa, base of tongue, supraglottic larynx, oropharynx, hypopharynx and nasopharynx is substantial.

In contrast, distant metastases from head and neck tumors are relatively uncommon. However, this may only reflect present limited ability to deal with advanced tumors. Patients may die of local disease before they can manifest distant disease. Merino et al.[105] recently reported a 10% overall incidence of distant spread.

Treatment of head and neck cancers requires close interdisciplinary cooperation. In general, either radiation therapy or surgery is capable of controlling early disease with equal efficacy.[106-108] This permits the patient and the patient's physicians to select therapy on the basis of cosmetic results and the patient's preference. A few sites, however, do predispose to a specific form of management. Carcinomas of the tip of the tongue can quickly and effectively be dealt with by surgery without causing either cosmetic or functional defect. Similarly carcinomas limited to the vocal cords, treated by radiotherapy, are likely to be cured without detriment to the quality of the voice.

Advanced lesions are controlled poorly either by surgery or radiotherapy. Surgery frequently fails because of the inability to encompass all of the tumor owing to the complex structure of the head and neck region. Radiation also fails, but for a different reason. Radiation can effectively deal with the peripheral tendrils of tumor; however, it is unable to control a bulky tumor with a hypoxic core, because of the limited radiosensitivity of hypoxic cells (Chap. 11). Because of the different modes of failure of surgery and radiotherapy, programs have evolved wherein modalities are combined. Whether radiation should be given preoperatively or postoperatively is an unsettled issue; however, it is clear that the combination is more effective than either modality alone and that morbidity resulting from combined procedures is acceptable.[109,110]

Since there is a substantial incidence of regional lymph node involvement, successful treatment of head and neck tumors usually includes therapy of the cervical nodes. When these nodes contain only subclinical amounts of tumor, moderate dose irradiation nearly always prevents subsequent tumor growth.[111] When clinically detectable tumor is present, surgical dissection frequently becomes necessary to avoid potential complications of high dose irradiation which would be necessary for hypoxic disease (Chap. 11). However, in such cases, combined surgery and moderate dose irradiation produces better local control than surgery alone[111] without producing undue morbidity.

Chemotherapeutic management of non-metastatic head and neck carcinomas, at present is experimental in nature. Borgelt and Davis[112] recently have reviewed the literature pertaining to the addition of chemotherapy to irradiation. Unfortunately, they found that single-agent adjuvant chemotherapy does not significantly alter survival, local control or the rate of development of distant metastases.

On the other hand, if symptomatic widespread metastases arise, chemotherapy can provide transient palliation. Lane et al.[113] produced objective responses which persisted for 4 months in 50% of patients treated with methotrexate. Bleomycin or cis-platinum either alone or in combination with methotrexate are also active against head and neck cancers.

Because of the wide variety of types of head and neck tumors, as well as individual variation secondary to the size of tumor, survival rates range from less than 10 to more than 90%. Far advanced local lesions with massive bilateral adenopathy, rarely, if ever, are cured. Small vocal cord cancers are associated with cure rates of 90 to 95%. Overall, when most common neoplasms and the usual range of sizes are considered, 5-year survival rates approximate 40 to 50%. As a basic "rule of thumb," when clinical adenopathy exists, survival rates approximately are halved.

Brain. Brain tumors form a unique group of lesions. None of the various types of brain tumors arise from neural cells. Rather, most arise from supporting glial cells. In adults, they are uncommon, accounting for only about 5% of all tumors. But, in children, they are the most common type of solid tumors and account for 20% of all cancers.

Histologic classification of brain tumors can be a source of confusion. A number of systems are in common use, and they differ somewhat. However, for most purposes, the following simplified concepts suffice. The majority of lesions derive from astrocytes. When all the tumor cells appear alike, the tumor is termed a well-differentiated or grade I astrocytoma. When cells are pleomorphic and mitotic rate is high, the tumor is called an anaplastic or grade IV astrocytoma or a glioblastoma multiforme. In adults, glioblastomas predominate, but, in children, well-differentiated astrocytomas are favored. Adults also have a substantial incidence of meningiomas, and children are prone to develop medulloblastomas. Other types of tumors such as ependymomas, oligodendrogliomas, pituitary adenomas, craniopharyngiomas and pineal tumors occur less commonly.

Clinically, approximately two-thirds of brain tumors in adults are supratentorial, in the cerebrum, while a similar proportion in children are infratentorial, in the cerebellum. The associated symptoms tend to reflect the precise site of origin. Each area of the brain controls specific functions, and tumors, by virtue of their presence, can inhibit or stimulate these functions. Lesions in the frontal region tend to alter personality and/or motor power; lesions in the parietal region, sensory functions; lesions in the temporal region, speech; lesions in the occipital region, vision and lesions in the cerebellum, coordination. In addition, tumors in any location can produce increased intracranial pressure which typically manifests as headache, vomiting and/or papilledema.

Brain tumors grow almost entirely by local extension. Within the brain, there are no barriers, and spread into more than one lobe or into the contralateral half of the brain is common. Concannon et al.[114] reviewed autopsy findings in patients who died of incidental causes shortly after having been diagnosed as having primary brain tumors. Despite clinical clues, skull x rays, angiography and radionuclide brain scans, the complete extent of tumor had been underestimated during life, in approximately 85% of cases. Although neoplastic cells can be dropped into the cerebrospinal fluid and thereby seed any part of the entire spinal cord, such spread is unusual, except in the medulloblastomas (and perhaps infratentorial tumors in general) where it is relatively common.

Lymph node metastases do not occur and the incidence of distant metastases is *very* small. Brain tumors, despite their localized nature, often fail to be treated successfully. The initial step in management should be surgical whenever feasible; however, the extent of resection must be tempered by the extreme risk of injuring normal brain tissue. Most often, only partial excision is possible. When the lesion is relatively inaccessible, surgery—other than a shunting procedure to decrease pressure—may not be warranted.

Because of the preceding factors, few cerebral tumors can be treated successfully by surgery alone. Notable exceptions are meningiomas in adults and well-differentiated cystic astrocytomas in the posterior fossae of children, both of which usually are controlled by surgery alone. However, in the majority of cases, radiotherapy should be called upon to aid in local therapy.

Fazekas[115] retrospectively analyzed treatment of *well*-differentiated astrocytomas. In grossly excised lesions, radiotherapy appeared unnecessary, but for all patients having incompletely excised tumors, adjuvant irradiation significantly improved survival. Sheline's series[116] supports the same conclusions.

Because of practical limitations which prevent total resection of nearly all *poorly*-differentiated gliomas and the aggressive biologic behavior of such lesions, radiotherapy is indicated for all glioblastomas. Prospective nationwide randomized trials[117] as well as retrospective series[116] have demonstrated the advantage in survival conferred by adjuvant irradiation.

In cases where surgery would be hazardous, radiation provides the primary form of management. Greenberger et al.[118] have recently reported their results of treatment of thalamic, mid-brain and brain-stem gliomas; tumors that rarely can be benefitted by surgery. Radiation produced an improvement in functional status in more than two-thirds of patients and disease free 1 to 5 or more year survivals in nearly one-half of all cases.

At present the role of chemotherapy is less clear. Prospective randomized trials suggest that the addition of a nitrosourea to surgery and irradiation increases survival of patients having anaplastic tumors;[117] however, the preferred drug, dose and indications for adjuvant chemotherapy in brain tumors has not yet been established. Survival after therapy for a brain tumor primarily is dependent upon histologic type and degree of differentiation of the lesion although feasibility of resection and adequacy of irradiation play important roles. For well-differentiated cystic astrocytomas of the cerebellum which are completely excised, survival is the rule. For incompletely excised better differentiated cerebral lesions treated by irradiation, 5-year disease free survivals in the range of 35 to 60%, depending on the precise degree of differentiation, are likely. Poorly differentiated lesions are associated with a 10 to 20% survival rate, and patients stricken by the most anaplastic tumor rarely, if ever, survive for 5 years.[115-117]

References

1. Klein, E., Case, R.W., and Burgess, G.H.: Chemotherapy of Skin Cancer. Ca—A Cancer Journal for Clinicians 23:228–231, 1973.
2. Clark, W.H., Jr., et al.: The Histogenesis and Biologic Behavior of Primary Human Malignant Melanomas of the Skin. Cancer Res. 29:705–727, 1969.
3. Breslow, A.: Thickness, Cross-Sectional Areas and Death of Invasion in The Prognosis of Cutaneous Melanoma. Ann. Surg. 172:902–908, 1970.
4. Mimh, M.C., Jr., Clark, W.H., and From, L.: The Clinical Diagnosis, Classification and Histogenetic Concepts of the Early Stages of Cutaneous Malignant Melanomas. N. Engl. J. Med. 284:1078–1082, 1971.
5. Gumport, S.L., and Harris, M.N.: Results of Regional Lymph Node Dissections for Melanoma. Ann. Surg. 179:105–108, 1974.
6. Cooper, J.S., Kopf, A.W., and Bart, R.S.: Present Role and Future Prospects for Radiotherapy in the Management of Malignant Melanomas. J. Dermatol. Surg. Oncol. 5:134–139, 1979.
7. Kopf, A.W., Bart, R.S., and Rodriguez-Sains, R.S.: Malignant Melanoma: A Review. J. Dermatol. Surg. Oncol. 3:4–125, 1977.
8. Eagan, R.T., et al.: Small Cell Carcinoma of the Lung: Staging, Paraneoplastic Syndromes, Treatment and Survival. Cancer 33:527–532, 1974.
9. Newman, S.J., and Hansen, H.H.: Frequency, Diagnosis and Treatment of Brain Metastases in 247 Consecutive Patients with Bronchogenic Carcinoma. Cancer 33:492–496, 1974.
10. Morrison, R.: The Treatment of Carcinoma of the Bronchus: A Clinical Trial to Compare Surgery and Supervoltage Radiotherapy. Lancet 1:683–684, 1963.

11. Boyd, D.P.: Is Extended Radical Resection Superior to Lobectomy in Treating Resectable Bronchial Cancer? J.A.M.A. *195*:1033, 1966.
12. Clifton, E.E.: The Criteria for Operability and Resectability in Lung Cancer. J.A.M.A. *195*:1031–1032, 1966.
13. Smart, J.: Can Lung Cancer be Cured? J.A.M.A. *195*:1034, 1966.
14. Deeley, T.J.: The Treatment of Carcinoma of the Bronchus. Br. J. Radiol. *40*:801–822, 1967.
15. Caldwell, W.L., and Bagshaw, M.A.: Indications for and Results of Irradiation of Carcinoma of the Lung. Cancer *22*:999–1004, 1968.
16. Guttmann, R.: The Role of Radiotherapy in Inoperable Carcinoma of the Lung. In Clark, R.L., Cumley, R.W., McCay, et al. (Ed.): *Oncology 1970: Proceedings of the 10th International Cancer Congress.* Chicago, Year Book Medical Publishers, 1971, Vol. 4, pp. 81–85.
17. Bloedorn, F.G., et al.: Preoperative Irradiation in Bronchogenic Carcinoma. A.J.R. *92*:77–87, 1964.
18. A Collaborative Study: Preoperative Irradiation of Cancer of the Lung: Preliminary Report of a Therapeutic Trial. Cancer *23*:419–429, 1969.
19. Carbone, P.P., et al.: Lung Cancer: Perspectives and Prospects. Ann. Intern. Med. *73*:1003–1024, 1970.
20. Paulson, D.L.: The Survival Rate in Superior Sulcus Tumors Treated by Presurgical Irradiation. J.A.M.A. *196*:342–343, 1966.
21. Bitran, J.D., et al.: Metastatic Non-Oat-Cell Bronchogenic Carcinoma. JAMA *240*:2743–2746, 1978.
22. Shields, T.W. et al.: Adjuvant Cancer Chemotherapy after Resection of Carcinoma of the Lung. Cancer *40*:2057–2062, 1977.
23. Miller, A.B., Fox, W., and Tall, R.: Five-Year Follow-up of the Medical Research Council Comparative Trial of Surgery and Radiotherapy for the Primary Treatment of Small-Celled or Oat Celled Carcinoma of the Bronchus. Lancet *2*:501–505, 1969.
24. Choi, C.H., and Carey, R.W.: Small Cell Anaplastic Carcinoma of Lung: Reappraisal of Current Management. Cancer *37*:2651–2657, 1976.
25. Einhorn, L.H. et al.: Long-Term Results in Combined-Modality Treatment of Small Cell Carcinoma of the Lung. Semin. Oncol. *5*:309–313, 1978.
26. Bunn, P.A., Nugent, J.L., and Matthews, M.J.: Central Nervous System Metastases in Small Cell Bronchogenic Carcinoma. Semin. Oncol. *5*:314–322, 1978.
27. Burkitt, D.P.: Epidemiology of Cancer of the Colon and Rectum. Cancer *28*:3–13, 1971.
28. Jackson, B.R.: Contemporary Management of Rectal Cancer. Cancer *40*:2365–2374, 1977.
29. Evans, J.T., et al.: Management and Survival of Carcinoma of the Colon: Results of a National Survey by the American College of Surgeons. Ann. Surg. *188*:716–720, 1978.
30. Turnbull, R.B. et al.: Cancer of the Colon: The Influence of the No Touch Isolation Technic on Survival Rates. Ann. Surg., *166*:420–427, 1967.
31. Butcher, H.R.: Carcinoma of the Rectum. Choice between Anterior Resection and Abdominal Perineal Resection of the Rectum. Cancer *28*:204–207, 1971.
32. Williams, I.G.: Radiotherapy of Carcinoma of the Rectum. In *Cancer of the Rectum,* (Ed.) Dukes, C. Edinburgh, E. and S. Livingston, 1960, pp. 210–219.
33. Wang, C.C., and Schulz, M.D.: The Role of Radiation Therapy in the Management of Carcinoma of the Sigmoid, Rectosigmoid and Rectum. Radiology *79*:1–5, 1962.
34. Whiteley, H.W. et al.: Radiation Therapy in the Palliative Management of

Patients with Recurrent Cancer of the Rectum and Colon. Surg. Clin. North Am. 49:381–387, 1969.

35. Rao, A.R. *et al.*: Effectiveness of Local Radiotherapy in Colorectal Carcinoma. Cancer 42:1082–1086, 1978.

36. Rider, W.D.: The 1975 Gordon Richards Memorial Lecture: Is the Miles Operation Really Necessary for the Treatment of Rectal Cancer: J. Can. Assoc. Radiol. 26:167–175, 1975.

37. Papillon, J.: Intracavitary Irradiation of Early Rectal Cancer for Cure: A Series of 186 Cases. Cancer 36:696–701, 1975.

38. Taylor, F.W.: Cancer of the Colon and Rectum: A Study of Routes of Metastases and Death. Surgery 52:305–308, 1962.

39. Cass, A.W., Million, R.R., and Pfaff, W.W.: Patterns of Recurrence Following Surgery Alone for Adenocarcinoma of the Colon and Rectum. Cancer 37:2861–2865, 1976.

40. Gunderson, L.L., and Sosin, H.: Areas of Failure Found at Reoperation (Second or Symptomatic Look) Following "Curative Surgery" for Adenocarcinoma of the Rectum: Clinicopathologic Correlation and Implications for Adjuvant Therapy. Cancer 34:1278–1292, 1974.

41. Kligerman, M.M.: Radiotherapy and Rectal Cancer. Cancer 39:896–900, 1977.

42. Moertel, C.G.: Current Concepts in Cancer: Chemotherapy of Gastrointestinal Cancer. N. Engl. J. Med. 299:1049–1052, 1978.

43. Baker, L.H. *et al.*: Phase III Comparison of the Treatment of Advanced Gastrointestinal Cancer with Bolus Weekly 5-Fu vs. Methyl-CCNU plus Bolus Weekly 5-Fu: A Southwest Oncology Group Study. Cancer 38:1–7, 1976.

44. Higgins, G.A. *et al.*: Adjuvant Chemotherapy in the Surgical Treatment of Large Bowel Cancer. Cancer 38:1461–1467, 1976.

45. Lane, N. *et al.*: Clinico-Pathologic Analysis of the Surgical Curability of Breast Cancers: A Minimum Ten-Year Study of a Personal Series. Ann. Surg. 153:483–498, 1961.

46. Moss, W.T., Brand, W.N. and Battifora, H.: *Radiation Oncology: Rationale, Technique, Results.* 4th ed. St. Louis, The C. V. Mosby Co., 1973, p. 305.

47. Fisher, B. *et al.*: Postoperative Radiotherapy in the Treatment of Breast Cancer: Results of NSABP Clinical Trial. Ann. Surg. 172:711–732, 1970.

48. Lucas, F.V., and Perez-Mesa, C.: Inflammatory Carcinoma of the Breast. Cancer 41:1595–1605, 1978.

49. Haagensen, C.D., and Stout, A.P.: Carcinoma of the Breast: Criteria of Operability. Ann. Surg., 118:859–870, 1032–1051, 1943.

50. Haagensen, C.D.: *Diseases of the Breast.* 2nd Ed. Philadelphia, W. B. Saunders Co., 1971, p. 628.

51. Prosnitz, L.R. *et al.*: Radiation Therapy as Initial Treatment for Early Stage Cancer of the Breast Without Mastectomy. Cancer 39:917–923, 1977.

52. Fletcher, G.H.: Reflections on Breast Cancer. Int. J. Rad. Oncol., Biol. Phys. 1:769–779, 1976.

53. Handley, R.S.: The Conservative Radical Mastectomy of Patey: 10-Year Results in 425 Patients. Breast; Diseases of the Breast 2:16–19, 1976.

54. McWhirter, R.: Should More Radical Treatment be Attempted in Breast Cancer? Am. J. Roentgenol. 92:3–13, 1964.

55. Fisher, B. *et al.*: Comparison of Radical Mastectomy with Alternative Treatments for Primary Breast Cancer: A First Report of Results from a Prospective Randomized Clinical Trial. Cancer 39:2827–2839, 1977.

56. Peters, M.V.: Cutting the "Gordian Knot" in Early Breast Cancer. Ann. R. Coll. Phys. Surg. Can. 8:187–192, 1975.

57. Fletcher, G.H., Montague, E., and Nelson, A.J.: Combination of Conservative Surgery and Irradiation for Cancer of the Breast. Radiology 126:216–222, 1976.
58. Pierquin, B., Baillet, F., and Wilson, J. F.: Radiation Therapy in the Management of Primary Breast Cancer. Am. J. Roentgenol. 127:645–648, 1976.
59. Harris, J.R., Levene, M.B., and Hellman, S.: The Role of Radiation Therapy in the Primary Treatment of Carcinoma of the Breast. Semin. Oncol. 5:403–416, 1978.
60. Fisher, B. et al.: L-Phenylalanine Mustard (L-PAM) in the Management of Primary Breast Cancer. N. Engl. J. Med. 292:117–122, 1975.
61. Bonadonna, G. et al.: Combination Chemotherapy as an Adjuvant Treatment in Operable Breast Cancer. N. Engl. J. Med. 294:405–410, 1976.
62. Bonadonna, G. et al.: Are Surgical Adjuvant Trials Altering the Course of Breast Cancer? Sem. Oncol. 5:450–464, 1978.
63. Alexander, P.: The Bogey of the Immuno-Suppressive Action of Local Radiotherapy. Int. J. Rad. Oncol., Biol. Phys. 1:369–371, 1976.
64. Vaeth, J.M. et al.: Radiotherapeutic Management of Locally Advanced Carcinoma of the Breast. Cancer 30:107–112, 1972.
65. Alderman, S.J.: Combination Teletherapy and Iridium Implantation in the Treatment of Locally Advanced Breast Cancer. Cancer 38:1936–1938, 1976.
66. Whitmore, W.F.: The Natural History of Prostatic Cancer. Cancer 32:1104–1112, 1973.
67. Owen, W.L.: Cancer of the Prostate: A Literature Review. J. Chron. Dis. 29:89–114, 1976.
68. Hanash, K.A. et al.: Carcinoma of the Prostate: A 15-year Followup. J. Urol. 107:450–453, 1972.
69. Grayhack, J.T., and Kripp, K.A.: Carcinoma of the Prostate. Urol. 2:1–16, 1975.
70. Bagshaw, M.A. et al.: External Beam Radiation Therapy of Primary Carcinoma of the Prostate. Cancer 36:723–728, 1975.
71. Hill, D.R., Crews, O.E., and Walsh, P.C.: Prostate Carcinoma: Radiation Treatment of the Primary and Regional Lymphatics. Cancer 34:156–160, 1974.
72. Perez, C.A. et al.: Radiation Therapy in the Definitive Treatment of Localized Carcinoma of the Prostate. Cancer 40:1425–1433, 1977.
73. Taylor, W.J.: Radiation Oncology: Cancer of the Prostate. Cancer 39:856–861, 1977.
74. Byar, D.P.: The Veterans Administration Cooperative Urological Research Group's Studies of Cancer of the Prostate. Cancer 32:1126–1130, 1973.
75. Moss, W.T., Brand, W.N., and Battifora, H.: Radiation Oncology: Rationale, Technique, Results, 4th Ed., St. Louis, The C. V. Mosby Co., 1973, p. 413.
76. Jampolis, S., Andras, E.J., and Fletcher, G.H.: Analysis of Sites and Causes of Failures of Irradiation in Invasive Squamous Cell Carcinoma of the Intact Uterine Cervix. Radiology 115:681–685, 1975.
77. Rousseau, J., et al.: Carcinoma of the Cervix: A 7-year Study of 1,212 Cases Treated at Fondation Curie, Paris. Radiology 103:413–418, 1972.
78. Brunschwig, A.: The Surgical Treatment of Cancer of the Cervix: Stage I and II. A.J.R. 102:147–151, 1968.
79. Symmonds, R.E.: Some Surgical Aspects of Gynecologic Cancer. Cancer 36:649–660, 1975.
80. dePalo, G.M. et al.: Methotrexate (NSC-740) and Bleomycin (NSC-125066) in the Treatment of Advanced Epidermoid Carcinoma of the Uterine Cervix. Cancer Chemother. Rep. 57:429–435, 1973.
81. Stolinksy, D.C., and Bateman, J.R.: Further Experience with Hexamethylamelamine (NSC 13875) in the Treatment of Carcinoma of the Cervix. Cancer Chemother. Rep. 57:497–499, 1973.

82. Morrow, C.P., DeSaia, P.J., and Townsend, D.E.: Current Management of En-
    dometrial Carcinoma. Obstet. Gynecol. *42*:399–406, 1973.
83. Moss, W.T., Brand, W.N., and Battifora, H.: *Radiation Oncology: Rationale,
    Technique, Results*. 4th Ed., St. Louis, The C. V. Mosby Co., 1973, p. 458.
84. Wharam, M.D., Phillips, T.L., and Bagshaw, M.: The Role of Radiation Therapy
    in Clinical Stage 1 Carcinoma of the Endometrium. Int. J. Rad. Oncol., Biol.
    Phys. *1*:1081–1089, 1976.
85. Salazar, O.M., et al.: The Management of Clinical Stage 1 Endometrial Car-
    cinoma. Cancer *41*:1016–1026, 1978.
86. Bruckman, J.E. et al.: Combined Irradiation and Surgery on the Treatment of
    Stage II Carcinoma of the Endometrium. Cancer *42*:1146–1151, 1978.
87. Antoniades, J., Brady, L.W., and Lewis, G.C.: The Management of Stage III
    Carcinoma of the Endometrium. Cancer *38*:1838–1842, 1976.
88. Landgren, R.C. et al.: Irradiation of Endometrial Cancer in Patients with Medical
    Contraindication to Surgery or with Unresectable Lesions. A.J.R. *126*:148–154,
    1976.
89. Malkasian, G.D.: Carcinoma of the Endometrium, Effect of Stage and Grade on
    Survival. Cancer *41*:996–1001, 1978.
90. DiSaia, P.J., Morrow, C.P., and Townsend, D.E.: *Synopsis of Gynecologic
    Oncology*. New York, John Wiley & Sons, 1975, pp. 113–135.
91. Bagley, C.M. et al.: Ovarian Carcinoma Metastatic to the Diaphragm—
    Frequently Undiagnosed at Laparotomy: A Preliminary Report. Am. J. Obstet.
    Gynecol. *116*:397–400, 1973.
92. Tobias, J.S., and Griffiths, C.T.: Management of Ovarian Carcinoma: Current
    Concepts and Future Prospects. N. Engl. J. Med. *294*:818–824, 877–882, 1976.
93. Hilaris, B.S., and Clark, D.G.C.: The Value of Postoperative Intraperitoneal
    Injection of Radiocolloids in Early Cancer of the Ovary. A.J.R. *112*:749–754,
    1971.
94. Delclos, L., and Quinlan, E.J.: Malignant Tumors of the Ovary Managed with
    Postoperative Megavoltage Irradiation. Radiology *93*:659–663, 1969.
95. Smith, J.P., and Rutledge, F.: Chemotherapy in the Treatment of Cancer of the
    Ovary. Am. J. Obstet. Gynecol. *107*:691–703, 1970.
96. Frick, H.C. et al.: Disseminated Carcinoma of the Ovary Treated by
    L-Phenylalanine Mustard. Cancer *21*:508, 1968.
97. Smith, J.P., and Rutledge, F.: Advances in Chemotherapy for Gynecologic
    Cancer. Cancer *36*:669–674, 1975.
98. Buchler, D.A. et al.: Stage III Ovarian Carcinoma: Treatment and Results.
    Radiology *122*:469–472, 1977.
99. Bush, R.S. et al.: Treatment of Epithelial Carcinoma of the Ovary: Operation,
    Irradiation, and Chemotherapy. Am. J. Obstet. Gynecol. *127*:692–704, 1977.
100. Fuks, Z., and Bagshaw, M.A.: The Rationale for Curative Radiotherapy for
     Ovarian Carcinoma. Int. J. Radiat. Oncol., Biol. Phys. *1*:21–32, 1975.
101. Flink, H. et al.: Maximal Radiation Therapy by a New Treatment Technique for
     Stage III Ovarian Cancer. Int. J. Radiat. Oncol., Biol. Phys. *4*:441–443, 1978.
102. Young, R.C. et al.: Advanced Ovarian Adenocarcinoma. N. Engl. J. Med.
     299:1261–1266, 1978.
103. Marchetta, F.C., Sako, K., and Camp, R.: Multiple Malignancies in Patients with
     Head and Neck Cancer. Am. J. Surg. *110*:537–541, 1965.
104. Lindberg, R.: Distribution of Cervical Lymph Node Metastases from Squamous
     Cell Carcinoma of the Upper Respiratory and Digestive Tracts. Cancer
     6:1446–1449, 1972.
105. Merino, O.R., Lindberg, R.D., and Fletcher, G.H.: An Analysis of Distant Metas-
     tases from Squamous Cell Carcinoma of the Upper Respiratory and Digestive
     Tracts. Cancer *40*:145–151, 1977.

106. Cocke, E.W., and Wang, C.C.S.: Cancer of the Larynx: Selecting Optimum Treatment. Ca—A Cancer Journal for Clinicians 26:194–200, 1976.

107. Cocke, E.W.: Cancer of the Larynx: Surgery. Ca—A Cancer Journal for Clinicians 26:201–211, 1976.

108. Wang, C.C.S.: Cancer of the Larynx: Radiation Therapy. Ca—A Cancer Journal for Clinicians 26:212–218, 1976.

109. Hamberger, A.D., et al.: Advanced Squamous Cell Carcinoma of the Oral Cavity and Oropharynx Treated with Irradiation and Surgery. Radiology 119:433–438, 1976.

110. Fletcher, G.H., and Jesse, R.H.: The Place of Irradiation in the Management of the Primary Lesion in Head and Neck Cancers. Cancer 39:862–867, 1977.

111. Jesse, R.H., and Fletcher, G.H.: Treatment of the Neck in Patients with Squamous Cell Carcinoma of the Head and Neck. Cancer 39:868–872, 1977.

112. Borgelt, B.B., and Davis, L.W.: Combination Chemotherapy and Irradiation for Head and Neck Cancer: A Review. Cancer Clin. Trials 1:49–59, 1978.

113. Lane, M., Moore, J.E., Levin, H., and Smith, F.E.: Methotrexate Therapy for Squamous Cell Carcinomas of the Head and Neck: Intermittent Intravenous Dose Program. J.A.M.A. 204:561–564, 1968.

114. Concannon, J.P., Kramer, S., and Berry, R.: The Extent of Intracranial Gliomata at Autopsy and its Relationship to Techniques used in Radiation Therapy of Brain Tumors. A.J.R., 84:99–107, 1960.

115. Fazekas, J.T.: Treatment of Grades I and II Brain Astrocytomas. The Role of Radiotherapy. Int. J. Radiat. Oncol., Biol. Phys. 2:661–666, 1977.

116. Sheline, G.E.: Radiation Therapy of Brain Tumors. Cancer 39:873–881, 1977.

117. Walsh, J.M., Cassady, J.R., Frei, E., Kornblith, P.L., and Welch, K.: Recent Advances in the Treatment of Primary Brain Tumors. Arch. Surg. 110:696–702, 1975.

118. Greenberger, J.S., Cassady, J.R., and Levene, M.B.: Radiation Therapy of Thalamic, Midbrain and Brain Stem Gliomas. Radiology 122:463–468, 1977.

3

WORK-UP AND
STAGING

Investigation of the extent of disease, commonly termed a staging work-up, must be a first step in logical oncologic management. Independent of the type of disease, the sites of involvement influence the objective of treatment and determine the methods which should be used. Cure of disease requires that all affected sites be treated, at the same time remembering that side effects and complications of therapy mandate that as few sites as possible be treated. Consequently, as a general rule, localized disease should be treated by local methods (either radiotherapy, surgery or regional chemotherapy). Of course, type and precise location of disease modify these basic plans but the more accurately extent of disease can be defined, the more likely the proposed treatment plan will be appropriate.

On the other hand, practical limitations to the extent of investigation that can be done exist. One cannot order every known test routinely. The time needed to perform many tests, the monetary expense and the risks and discomfort of at least some demand that a rational approach to work-up be taken.

The purpose of this chapter is to discuss various tests commonly used in a staging work-up, their advantages and disadvantages, and provide a general philosophy of their use. Subsequently, the ten types of tumor discussed in Chapter 2 are reviewed in terms of factors which influence staging, and guidelines for work-up are recommended.

General Principles. Appropriate work-up is a rationally devised plan which maximizes chance of therapeutic success but minimizes patients' risks. Appropriate tests contribute to the determination of extent of disease, provide information which may alter treatment planning and are the least invasive and/or expensive ways of obtaining this information. The first requirement demands that the physician be intimately familiar with the natural history and biologic behavior of the disease in question. Every disease has a characteristic mode of spread, and work-up specifically should be directed toward frequent target areas of the body. In addition, when the chance of spread of disease to a particular site is relatively small, but the importance of discovering disease in that site is great, tests should be done to investigate this possibility. Last, if two procedures are equally likely to yield the same information, the procedure with the lesser risk of morbidity should be chosen. If two procedures are in all other respects similar, the least expensive means should be used.

The Work-up. Work-up conveniently can be considered in four categories: (1) basic tests done for all patients, (2) specialized laboratory tests, (3) specialized radiographic procedures and (4) specialized diagnostic surgical procedures.

Basic Tests. History and physical examinations obviously are vital to care of any patient. Devoid of risk, they provide a fairly accurate picture of extent of disease. Preferably, both history and physical examination should be directed toward tumor related information. For the patient who does not have an established diagnosis, etiologic factors should be sought. For example, a middle aged man who develops a cough and has a long standing history of heavy tobacco use is a prime candidate for bronchogenic carcinoma. On the other hand, a similar patient who worked in an industry where he was exposed to asbestos, needs be considered possibly to have a mesothelioma. At times, the chronology of the patient's symptoms can be a clue to the site of disease. For example, a patient who complains of hoarseness and difficulty swallowing may prove to have a tumor in his larynx or pharynx. If hoarseness preceded difficulty in swallowing, statistics favor a laryngeal primary, whereas if difficulty in swallowing preceded hoarseness, a hypopharyngeal primary is favored.

Similarly an understanding of mode of tumor spread can help direct physical examination. For example, a middle aged man who develops cough and hoarseness after many years of cigarette use merely may be reacting to irritation of his upper respiratory tract mucosa, may have a primary tumor of his larynx with a "smoker's cough" or may have a primary bronchogenic carcinoma which has invaded his left recurrent laryngeal nerve, fixing his left vocal cord in the midline position. Indirect laryngoscopy quickly will distinguish between these possibilities. Or to present another example, a female with an advanced gynecologic malignancy readily may be found to have distant disease during a careful examination of her left supraclavicular fossa. The preceding comments should not be taken as our approval of anything less than a thorough physical for every patient; however, a knowledge of tumor behavior will permit the physician to direct his attention to specific sites which might otherwise be overlooked.

A complete blood count is relatively inexpensive and devoid of side effects. It too should be part of every routine work-up. Decreased hemoglobin values impair the efficacy of radiotherapy (Chap. 11), decreased white blood cell or platelet counts make chemotherapeutic management difficult (Chap. 5).

Serum electrolytes and basic liver and kidney function tests, inexpensively done as part of an SMA-12 series, are without risks and provide a basic chemistry screen. Electrolytes may disclose a paraneoplastic syndrome (Chap. 15), liver function tests may detect metastases from a variety of sources and renal function tests are imperative with certain tumors which may obstruct the urinary tract, such as cervical neoplasms.

Another test which can be advocated routinely is a chest x-ray. It entails little risk and is relatively inexpensive. On the other hand, it may detect pulmonary metastases and, equally important, may disclose a co-existent pulmonary pathologic condition which may alter the physician's ability to work-up or treat a patient in a "standard" fashion. For example, a patient with carcinoma of the cervix who has severe non-neoplastic pulmonary pathology should not have a lymphangiogram.

Biopsy. Biopsy confirmation of tumor is essential in nearly all cases. In addition to proving the existence of cancer, biopsy can identify type of tumor cell, probable tissue of origin, degree of differentiation, depth of invasion and likely subsequent behavior. All of these factors modify required management, as will be discussed in the following chapters. Thus, few situations justify omitting a biopsy; however, some exceptions do exist.

Exceptions basically are limited to situations wherein biopsy would be hazardous and the clinical picture strongly suggests a neoplastic etiology. An adult who suddenly experiences severe headaches, nausea, vomiting and visual disturbances and has a single area of abnormal uptake in the region of the thalamus on a brain scan and/or a computerized tomogram should be accepted as having a thalamic brain tumor without biopsy.

Furthermore, a biopsy which fails to disclose tumor should not be interpreted as proof that a tumor does not exist. Injudicious selection of biopsy site may miss the lesion and detect only host reaction to the tumor. At times, persistent repetitive sampling is necessary to detect a tumor when the clinical picture and histologic findings seem incompatible. For example, patients who eventually are found to have a lymphoma of the skin frequently relate a history of having had multiple previous biopsies of clinically similar lesions, which only demonstrated "inflammation." In such cases, providing the pathologist with a clinical synopsis not infrequently can aid him in arriving at the correct histologic interpretation.

Thus, the biopsy must be viewed just as one more, albeit powerful, test in the work-up of cancer.

The optimal method of biopsy deserves discussion because, in essence, there is none. The preferred type of biopsy in a given case depends upon the clinical situation including size, type, location and accessibility of tumor.

Two basic methods of biopsy exist: excisional and incisional. An excisional biopsy removes all clinically evident tumor, but an incisional biopsy removes only a part. When the lesion occupies an accessible space and can be encompassed by a simple surgical procedure, excisional biopsy should be performed. However, a degree of surgical expertise is required even for such simple procedures to prevent subsequent difficulties. For example, current recommendations for surgical management of cutaneous melanomas include re-excision of the biopsy site, and removal of any remaining tumor and wide borders of clinically uninvolved skin. To produce such large margins without requiring extensive skin grafts to cover the defect, the surgeon utilizes the natural mobility of the skin. A biopsy done without regard to the directions in which skin can be moved can substantially complicate subsequent surgery.

In all other cases, incisional biopsy is preferred and several subtypes of incisional biopsy are in common use. A scalpel can be used to slice a biopsy from either the side or top of a lesion, a "punch" can be used to core out a somewhat cylindrical piece of tissue or a wide bore needle can be used to remove a fragment of a tumor which is deep inside an organ (Fig. 3–1). Whatever method is used, a representative sample should be sought to provide the pathologist as much aid as possible.

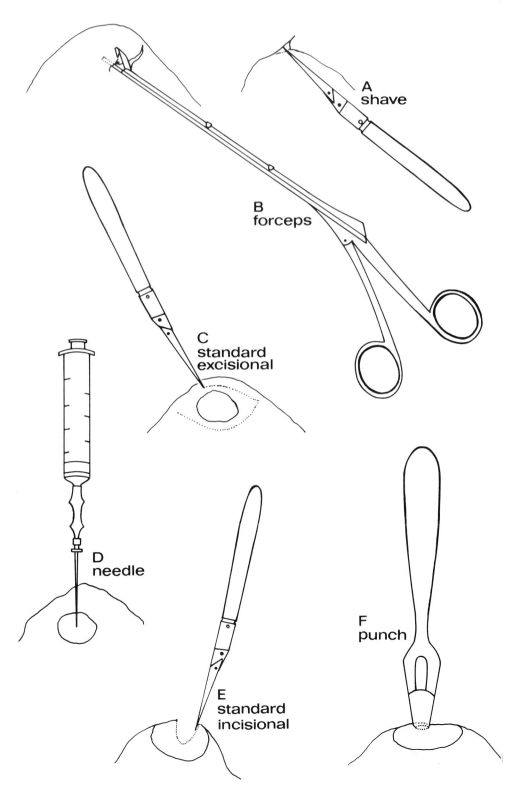

A
shave

B
forceps

C
standard
excisional

D
needle

E
standard
incisional

F
punch

Fig. 3–1. *Methods of biopsy.*

Special Laboratory Tests. These should be ordered only when previous work-up indicates that they are likely to provide essential information. Although they cause minimal morbidity, their expense can be considerable and, in unselected patients, they are not likely to improve the quality of medical care. A wide variety of tests fall into this category, and the principles these tests are based upon varies. As yet, the perfect test to detect cancer, particularly in its earliest stages, does not exist. However, some types of tumors sometimes are associated with specific markers in the patient's serum. Cancers in the gastrointestinal tract sometimes liberate a specific substance, carcinoembryonic antigen, normally detectable only in fetal life. Some testicular tumors are associated with elevated levels of human chorionic gonadotrophin and/or alpha-fetoprotein. Advanced prostatic carcinomas usually produce abnormally high acid phosphatase levels. Recently, Podolsky *et al.*[1] described the utility of galactosyltransferase isoenzyme II as a general marker. In 165 of 232 cases having diverse types of cancer, this isoenzyme was detectable. Unfortunately, these tests are not always positive in the presence of neoplastic disease and sometimes are elevated in the absence of neoplastic disease for other reasons. Perhaps the best conclusion to draw is that these tests are helpful, but not infallible. One interesting variation on this theme occurs in patients who have medullary thyroid tumors. Approximately 80% of such patients have elevated levels of thyrocalcitonin in their serum; after calcium is infused, nearly all patient's sera are positive for thyrocalcitonin. Thus, in certain circumstances, detection of tumor markers can be stimulated.

At other times special lab tests can detect sites of tumor involvement by changes produced in affected organs. For example, a bronchogenic carcinoma causing an elevated alkaline phosphatase level is likely to have metastasized to bone or liver or both. If the 5'nucleotidase level is normal, disease is probably in bone, but if it is elevated, disease is in liver (and maybe bone too).

Last, there are tests that detect changes distant from the tumor. Active Hodgkin's disease frequently produces an increase in the erythrocyte sedimentation rate, an increase in the serum copper level and a decrease in the serum zinc level.

Radiographs. Diagnostic radiographs rely upon differences in atomic number to differentiate between tissues. As a result, because tumors are structurally similar in this regard to normal tissues, non-contrast radiographs usually will not demonstrate tumors directly.

However, when tumors are adjacent to air filled spaces, they may be apparent. For example, a large lesion of the base of the tongue may be seen as an irregular mass in the distorted oropharyngeal air space on a lateral film. Less commonly, a tumor will stand out because of an unusual intrinsic property. An osteogenic sarcoma, because of its high density, may show up in contrast to the surrounding soft tissue, just as a liposarcoma, because of its relatively low density may be apparent against tissue of the retroperitoneum.

Tumors which metastasize to bone may change the osseous architecture and, therefore, be apparent. Most frequently, a dissolution of bone occurs and a less dense, or lytic, region appears on the film. Many types of tumors produce this type of change, the most common being breast and lung. Unfortunately, by the time lytic lesions become

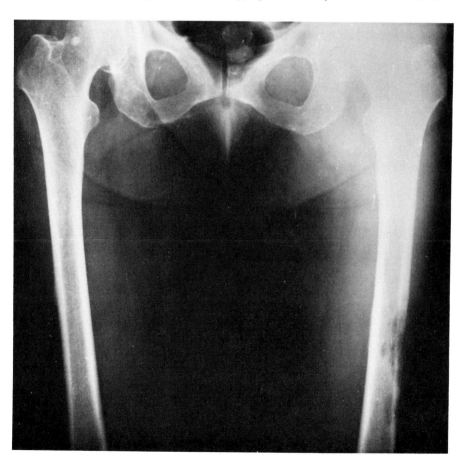

Fig. 3—2. *Example of lytic metastasis.*

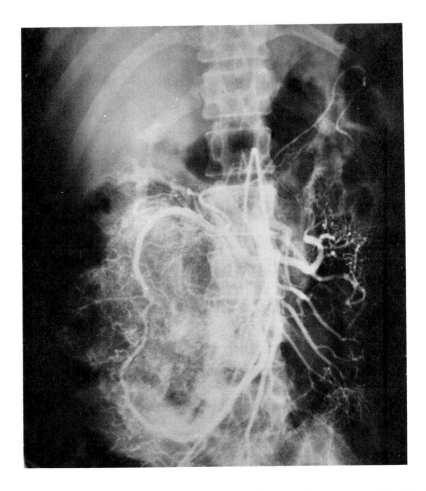

Fig. 3–4. *Angiogram demonstrating neovascularity of mesenteric sarcoma in right side of abdomen.*

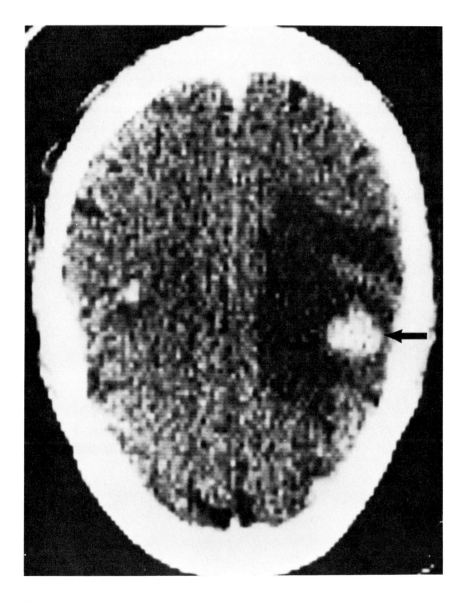

Fig. 3–5.   *Contrast enhanced computerized tomogram of brain. Arrow indicates lesion (light area) with surrounding edema (dark area).*

Radionuclide Scans. Radionuclide scans detect the disintegrations of various radioactive isotopes which can be administered to patients. Certain parts of the body attract those isotopes and using the radiations emanating from the isotope, specific organs or parts can be imaged. In some sites increased uptake of the isotope indicates disease. This is true of a bone scan where increased bone turnover will increase the pick-up rate of the radioisotope. In other sites, decreased uptake indicates disease. Destruction of hepatic parenchyma by tumor will prevent uptake of isotope in that region. Scans are considerably more sensitive in detecting disease than are x rays; however, they are less selective. Thus, a patient who has increased activity in a limited number of sites on a bone scan must have ordinary x rays of the affected area to rule out benign causes (such as osteoarthritis).

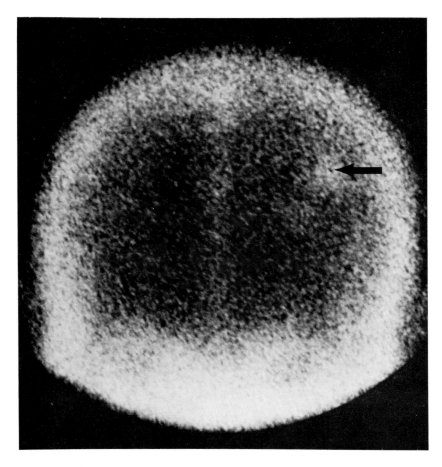

Fig. 3–6. *Brain scan. Arrow indicates lesion (increased uptake).*

Surgery. Diagnostic surgery currently plays a vital role in management of some types of tumor. In critical sites, where noninvasive methods cannot be used to evaluate the presence or absence of disease, biopsy can provide irrefutable evidence of tumor. On the other hand, risks inherent in any surgical procedure demand that such procedures be reserved for situations wherein the demonstration of tumor would substantially alter the plan of treatment.

The prototype of surgical work-up is the staging laparotomy as is used for Hodgkin's disease. By this procedure, histopathologic examination of representative samples from lymph nodes, liver and bone marrow, as well as the entire spleen, is possible. In other circumstances, percutaneous routes provide access to many organs. Blind biopsy of bone marrow is a standard procedure for assessment of the leukemias, lymphomas, pediatric tumors and oat cell bronchogenic carcinomas. Directed hepatic biopsy can clarify equivocal liver scans or ultrasonograms, while fluoroscopically guided "skinny needle" biopsy appears to provide sufficient tissue for cytologic analysis from nearly any site in the body.

Last, surgery in the form of multiple blind biopsies may be required to discover the site of origin of head and neck tumors that present as a cervical lymph node mass without an obvious primary source.

Staging. Once established, knowledge of the extent of disease can be used as a guide to appropriate therapy, or afterwards, to compare the results of therapy obtained in similar patients. To facilitate such use, standard expressions of extent have been developed by several groups and termed, *staging criteria.* Over the course of time these criteria have been modified to conform with current concepts and the criteria vary somewhat from group to group. Thus, various staging systems may be applied to a given lesion with slightly different results. In addition, the methods of staging depend on anatomic site of origin. Some tumors are staged on clinical data, some radiographic data, and some require surgical data. For example, intra-oral tumors primarily are staged by physical examination; testicular tumors require radiographic investigation; and ovarian tumors cannot be staged without a surgical procedure. For some tumors, both clinical and surgical staging is permitted. Hodgkin's disease always can be staged clinically, but cases which have had a laparotomy also can be staged on histopathologic grounds and the clinical and pathologic stages need not agree. Because surgical staging more accurately determines the true extent of disease, the two types of staging cannot be compared and the pathologic stage frequently exceeds the clinical stage.

Staging Criteria. Although precise rules for staging tumors differ for each different type of tumor, some basic concepts apply universally. Stages usually are designated by Roman numerals ranging from one to four. Stage I represents the earliest manifestations of localized disease, stage IV usually denotes dissemination. In some cases, the size of the primary lesion determines the stage. In others, the depth of invasion and, in still others, the specific locations invaded by the primary tumor define the stage.

For some types of tumors, subclassification according to the extent of the primary tumor, involvement of lymph nodes and distant metastases is possible. Such systems designate *tumor size* by four categories of progressively increasing extent (i.e. T1, T2, T3, T4), *nodal extent* by four categories (i.e. N0 (no nodes), N1, N2, N3) and the absence or presence of *distant metastases* by two categories (i.e. M0 (no metastases), M1). Philosophically, staging aims to group lesions having a similar prognosis. Because different lesions exhibit different biologic behaviors, the factors which influence prognosis differ. Thus, staging rules are *specific* for the type of tumor. The balance of this chapter discusses the particular factors of importance for each of the previously discussed tumors, lists the specific staging criteria for them and finally, recommends *minimum* work-up needed to stage them accurately.

Staging Basics. In all cases, a basic work-up consisting of a complete history and physical examination, complete blood count, serum enzyme studies (SMA-12 or equivalent), chest x ray, and biopsy should be done. Additional minimum work-up required depends on the specific tumor type.

STAGING BY TUMOR TYPE

Skin Cancer. Staging of skin cancer[2] primarily is based on clinical data and the rules are listed in Table 3–1. Primary tumor extent basically is judged by the maximum diameter of the lesion. In addition, the depth of invasion uncovered by a diagnostic biopsy can advance the stage; however, this implies that the deepest extent of tumor has been found. Such staging rules, therefore, better apply to already resected lesions, i.e., postsurgical staging.

Work-up for a basal or squamous cell cancer need not be extensive. Indeed, the basic examination including careful inspection and palpation provides as much data as are usually needed. However, when lesions are solidly attached to underlying bony structures, x rays of the

Table 3–1. Staging of Cancer of the Skin[2]

Primary Tumor (T)

TIS	Preinvasive carcinoma (carcinoma *in situ*)
T0	No primary tumor present
T1	Tumor 2 cm or less in its largest dimension, strictly superficial or exophytic
T2	Tumor more than 2 cm but not more than 5 cm in the largest dimension or with minimal infiltration of the dermis, irrespective of size
T3	Tumor more than 5 cm in its largest dimension or with deep infiltration of the dermis, irrespective of size
T4	Tumor involving other structures such as cartilage, muscle, or bone

Nodal Involvement (N)

The nodal involvement for cervical nodes is identical to that of the head and neck cancers, and this can also be applied to other nodal regions as well.

N0		No clinically positive nodes
N1		Single clinically positive homolateral node less than 3 cm in diameter
N2		Single clinically positive homolateral node 3 to 6 cm in diameter or multiple clinically positive homolateral nodes, none over 6 cm in diameter
	N2a	Single clinically positive homolateral node 3 to 6 cm in diameter
	N2b	Multiple clinically positive homolateral nodes, none over 6 cm in diameter
N3		Massive homolateral node(s), bilateral nodes, or contralateral node(s)
	N3a	Clinically positive homolateral node(s), over 6 cm in diameter
	N3b	Bilateral clinically positive nodes (in this situation, each side of the neck should be staged separately; that is N3b: right, N2a; left N1)
	N3c	Contralateral clinically positive node(s) only

Distant Metastasis (M)

MX	Not assessed
MO	No (known) distant metastasis
M1	Distant metastasis present
	Specify _____

area should be done to rule out osseous involvement. Large recurrent lesions may give rise to pulmonary metastases sufficiently frequently that in such cases a chest x ray must be obtained.

Lung. Carcinoma of the lung basically is staged on radiographic criteria.[2] As can be seen in Table 3–2, both size of the primary lesion and its position are important because lesions close to the tracheal carina cannot be resected.

Table 3–2.   Staging of Pulmonary Carcinoma[2]

TNM CLASSIFICATION

Primary Tumor (T)

TX	Tumor proven by the presence of malignant cells in bronchopulmonary secretions but not visualized roentgenographically or bronchoscopically, or any tumor that cannot be assessed
T0	No evidence of primary tumor
TIS	Carcinoma in situ
T1	Tumor 3.0 cm or less in greatest diameter, surrounded by lung or visceral pleura, and without evidence of invasion proximal to a lobar bronchus at bronchoscopy.
T2	Tumor more than 3.0 cm in greatest diameter, or a tumor of any size that either invades the visceral pleura or has associated atelectasis or obstructive pneumonitis extending to the hilar region. At bronchoscopy the proximal extent of demonstrable tumor must be within a lobar bronchus or at least 2.0 cm distal to the carina. Any associated atelectasis or obstructive pneumonitis must involve less than an entire lung and there must be no pleural effusion
T3	Tumor of any size with direct extension into an adjacent structure such as the parietal pleura or the chest wall, the diaphragm, or the mediastinum and its contents; or a tumor demonstrable bronchoscopically to involve a main bronchus less than 2.0 cm distal to the carina; or any tumor associated with atelectasis or obstructive pneumonitis of an entire lung or pleural effusion

Nodal Involvement (N)

N0	No demonstrable metastasis to regional lymph nodes
N1	Metastasis to lymph nodes in the peribronchial or the ipsilateral hilar region, or both, including direct extension
N2	Metastasis to lymph nodes in the mediastinum

Distant Metastasis (M)

MX	Not assessed
MO	No (known) distant metastasis
M1	Distant metastasis present

Specify _____

Specify sites according to the following notations:

Pulmonary—PUL
Osseous—OSS
Hepatic—HEP
Brain—BRA
Lymph Nodes—LYM
Bone Marrow—MAR
Pleura—PLE
Skin—SKI
Eye—EYE
Other—OTH

STAGE GROUPING

Occult stage	TX	NO	MO	Occult carcinoma with bronchopulmonary secretions containing malignant cells but without other evidence of metastasis to the regional lymph nodes or distant metastasis

Table 3–2. (Cont'd)

Stage I	TIS	NO	MO	Carcinoma in situ
	T1	NO	MO	Tumor that can be classified T1 without any
	T1	N1	MO	metastasis or with metastasis to the lymph nodes
	T2	NO	MO	in the peribronchial and/or ipsilateral hilar region only or a tumor that can be classified T2 without any metastasis to nodes or distant metastasis
Stage II	T2	N1	MO	Tumor classified as T2 with metastasis to the lymph nodes in the peribronchial and/or ipsilateral hilar region only
Stage III	T3 with any N or M			Any tumor more extensive than T2, or any
	N2 with any T or M			tumor with metastasis to the lymph nodes
	M1 with any T or N			in the mediastinum, or any tumor with distant metastasis

Obviously, a chest x ray done in both the posterior-anterior and lateral positions is a particularly essential part of the work-up. The recent development of computerized tomographic equipment which has the ability to scan the thorax, now permits more accurate demarcation of disease than was previously possible. Because of the likelihood of distant metastases, all patients with bronchogenic carcinomas should also have a thorough investigation of the liver and skeletal system. Serum liver chemistries, with or without a liver scan, will suffice for the former and a bone scan with correlative x rays of areas of increased activity, are recommended for the latter. All patients having small cell (oat cell) tumors should, in addition, undergo brain scan and a bone marrow biopsy. If there is any question of the patient's overall pulmonary capacity, pulmonary function tests should be done to evaluate ability to tolerate treatment. If surgical therapy is being considered, mediastinoscopy becomes mandatory to detect nonresectable cases.

Colorectal Cancer. Staging of colorectal cancers is based upon degree of invasion of the primary tumor according to the commonly used Astler-Coller modification of Duke's staging system.[3] The precise criteria are listed in Table 3–3. Because the depth of invasion can only be accurately determined once the affected area is in the pathologist's laboratory, staging is postsurgical.

Investigation of colorectal tumors relies upon barium enema x rays and sigmoidoscopy to delimit the intraluminal extent of disease. For

Table 3–3. Staging of Colorectal Cancer[3]

A	Primary lesion limited to the mucosa
B₁	Primary lesion extending into but not through the muscular layer without lymph node involvement
B₂	Primary lesion extending through the muscular layer without lymph node involvement
C₁	Primary lesion confined within bowel wall with lymph node involvement
C₂	Primary lesion extending through the bowel wall with lymph node involvement

anteriorly placed lesions, cystoscopy should be done to rule out bladder involvement. Liver scans may be used as an adjunct to serum chemistries because of the substantial frequency of hepatic involvement. In addition, serum carcinoembryonic antigen levels, as a baseline for serial follow-up studies are necessary. At the time of surgery, thorough intra-abdominal exploration should precede resection.

Table 3–4. Staging of Breast Cancer[2]

TNM CLASSIFICATION
  Primary Tumor (T)
  Clinical-Diagnostic Classification

TX		Tumor cannot be assessed
T0		No evidence of primary tumor
TIS		Paget's disease of the nipple with no demonstrable tumor
		Note: Paget's disease with a demonstrable tumor is classified according to size of tumor
T1*		Tumor 2 cm or less in greatest dimension
	T1a	No fixation to underlying pectoral fascia or muscle
	T1b	Fixation to underlying pectoral fascia and/or muscle
T2*		Tumor more than 2 cm but not more than 5 cm in its greatest dimension
	T2a	No fixation to underlying pectoral fascia and/or muscle
	T2b	Fixation to underlying pectoral fascia and/or muscle
T3*		Tumor more than 5 cm in its greatest dimension
	T3a	No fixation to underlying pectoral fascia and/or muscle
	T3b	Fixation to underlying pectoral fascia and/or muscle
T4		Tumor of any size with direct extension to chest wall or skin
		Note: Chest wall includes ribs, intercostal muscles, and serratus anterior muscle, but not pectoral muscle
	T4a	Fixation to chest wall
	T4b	Edema (including peau d'orange), ulceration of the skin of the breast, or satellite skin nodules confined to the same breast
	T4c	Both of above
	T4d	Inflammatory carcinoma

* Dimpling of the skin, nipple retraction, or any other skin changes except those in T4b may occur in T1, T2, or T3 without changing the classification.

Table 3–4.   (Cont'd)

Nodal Involvement (N)
Clinical-Diagnostic Classification
NX   Regional lymph nodes cannot be assessed clinically
NO   No palpable homolateral axillary nodes
N1   Movable homolateral axillary nodes
    N1a   Nodes not considered to contain growth
    N1b   Nodes considered to contain growth
N2   Homolateral axillary nodes considered to contain growth and fixed
            to one another or to other structures
N3   Homolateral supraclavicular or infraclavicular nodes considered to
            contain growth or edema of the arm*

M—DISTANT METASTASIS
MX Not assessed
MO No (known) distant metastasis
M1 Distant metastasis present
    Specify _____
Specify sites according to the following notations:
            Pulmonary—PUL
            Osseous—OSS
            Hepatic—HEP
            Brain—BRA
        Lymph Nodes—LYM
        Bone Marrow—MAR
            Pleura—PLE
            Skin—SKI
            Eye—EYE
            Other—OTH

STAGE GROUPING

Stage	T	N	M
Stage I	T1a	NO or N1a	
	T1b	NO or N1a	MO
Stage II	T1	N1b	
	T2a	NO or N1a or N1b	
	T2b	NO or N1a or N1b	MO
Stage III	Any T3	N1 or N2	MO
Stage IV	T4	Any N	Any M
	Any T	N3	Any M
	Any T	Any N	M1

* Edema of the arm may be caused by lymphatic obstruction and lymph nodes may not then be palpable.

Breast. Carcinoma of the breast is staged primarily on clinical grounds.[2] The precise criteria are listed in Table 3–4, and, as can be seen, depend upon size of the lesion, the absence or presence of its fixation and the type of skin involvement.

In addition to biopsy for histologic diagnosis, all biopsies of breast cancer should be submitted for estrogen and progesterone receptor protein analysis (Chap. 6) as an aid for potential future management.

Mammography, including the contralateral breast, should be done because of the substantial incidence of multiple primary tumors. In addition, distant spread, most commonly to lungs (chest x ray), liver (chemistries, with or without scan) and bone (scan), needs to be ruled out. Although brain metastases from breast carcinoma occur relatively frequently, scans in asyptomatic patients are not routinely warranted. If there is any question about the patient's mental status, a computerized axial tomographic and/or a radionuclide brain scan should be ordered.

Table 3–5. Staging of Prostatic Tumors[2]

TNM CLASSIFICATION
Primary Tumor (T)

TO	No tumor palpable: includes incidental findings of a cancer in a biopsy or operative specimen
T1	Tumor intracapsular surrounded by normal gland
T2	Tumor confined to gland, deforming contour, and invading capsule, but lateral sulci and seminal vesicles are not involved
T3	Tumor extends beyond capsule with or without involvement of lateral sulci and/or seminal vesicles
T4	Tumor fixed or involving neighboring structures.
	Add suffix (m) after "T" to indicate multiple tumors (e.g., T2m)

Nodal Involvement (N)

NX	Minimum requirements cannot be met
N0	No involvement of regional lymph nodes
N1	Involvement of a single regional lymph node
N2	Involvement of multiple regional lymph nodes
N3	Free space between tumor and fixed pelvic wall mass
N4	Involvement of juxta-regional nodes

Note: If N category is determined by lymphangiography or isotope scans, insert "1" or "i" between "N" and appropriate numbers (e.g., N12 or Ni2). If nodes are histologically positive after surgery, add "+"; if negative, add "–".

Distant Metastasis (M)

MX	Not assessed
M0	No (known) distant metastasis
M1	Distant metastasis present
	Specify _____

Specify sites according to the following notations:

Pulmonary—PUL
Osseous—OSS
Hepatic—HEP
Brain—BRA
Lymph Nodes—LYM
Bone Marrow—MAR
Pleura—PLE
Skin—SKI
Eye—EYE
Other—OTH

Prostate. Carcinoma of the prostate is staged on clinical criteria (as shown in Table 3–5) basically on the findings of rectal examination.[2] Carcinoma of the prostate is unique in that elevated serum acid phosphatase levels may be viewed as an indication of advanced disease.

Staging of prostatic carcinoma presents a problem because the lymph nodes at risk are relatively inaccessible. A lymphangiogram will demonstrate only some of the nodes at risk, computerized axial tomography will not detect minute involvement and diagnostic surgical sampling requires an operative procedure. Thus, while these procedures have their advocates, they cannot be considered essential. On the other hand, distant metastases to bone should be ruled out by radionuclide scans, and an evaluation of local extension by cystoscopic and intravenous urographic x-ray examinations is mandatory.

Uterine Cervix. Staging of carcinoma of the cervix is based on physical and radiographic data as listed in Table 3–6.[2] Extent of disease and precise areas involved, in general, determine the stage. In addition, hydroureter is presumed to be secondary to neoplastic infiltration of the parametria, with consequent obstruction of the distal ureters, and the findings of hydroureter therefore places patients in the same stage as does advanced parametrial disease.

Biopsy of cervical carcinomas can be done by the punch method. When no lesion is grossly visible, the cervix face should be painted with Schiller's iodine stain. The glycogen of normal cervical mucosal cells will take up stain, but a tumor will not. Poorly stained areas are therefore suspicious for malignancy and warrant biopsy investigation.

Table 3–6. Staging of Cervical Carcinoma[2]

CERVIX UTERI			
Stage	0	(TIS)	Carcinoma in situ
Stage	I	(T1)	Carcinoma confined to cervix
	IA	(T1a)	Microinvasive carcinoma
	IB	(T1b)	All other cases of Stage I
Stage	II	(T2)	Carcinoma extends beyond cervix but not to pelvic wall or lower vagina
	IIA	(T2a)	No obvious parametrial involvement
	IIB	(T2b)	Obvious parametrial involvement
Stage	III	(T3)	Cancer extends to pelvic wall or lower vagina, or ureteral obstruction
	IIIA	(T3a)	No extension to pelvic wall
	IIIB	(T3b)	Extension to one or both pelvic walls, or ureteral obstruction
Stage	IV	(T4)	Carcinoma beyond true pelvis or invading bladder or rectum
	IVA	(T4a)	Spread to adjacent organs
	IVB	(T4b)	Spread to distant organs

Work-up of cervical carcinomas requires that an intravenous urogram be done to rule out hydroureter. In addition, this procedure will prevent the unwitting irradiation of a pelvic horseshoe kidney and may alert surgeons to pre-existing renal or uroteric pathologic condition prior to any contemplated surgery. Although yield will be low in early stage disease (and consequently the procedures may be omitted), cystoscopy, sigmoidoscopy (± barium enema x rays) should be done for all advanced lesions. Lymphangiography can be considered an optional procedure which at times provides much useful information. We advise its routine use for all but the earliest stage cases.

Uterine Endometrium. Carcinoma of the endometrium is staged on clinical grounds, and the precise rules are listed in Table 3–7.[2] As can be seen, these criteria are based on the location of the areas involved by tumor. In addition, while not part of the staging system, depth of invasion into the myometrium and histologic grade of the tumor are important factors in determining both treatment and prognosis.

Biopsy evidence of disease usually requires dilatation of the cervical *os* and curettage of the endometrial walls (D&C). To rule out extension to cervix (stage II disease), the cervix should be curettaged before a sample is taken from the endometrium (fractional D&C).

Because carcinoma of the uterus tends to be confined to the uterus for prolonged periods, an extensive work-up usually is not productive. However, an intravenous urogram is essential as a guide for the surgeon, and cystoscopy and sigmoidoscopy are recommended for advanced cases.

Ovarian Carcinoma. As can be seen in Table 3–8, the staging rules of ovarian carcinoma depend upon sites of involvement.[2] Because

Table 3–7.   Staging of Endometrial Carcinoma[2]

CORPUS UTERI			
Stage	0	(TIS)	Carcinoma in situ
Stage	I	(T1)	Carcinoma confined to the corpus
	IA	(T1a)	Uterine cavity 8 cm or less in length
	IB	(T1b)	Uterine cavity greater than 8 cm in length
Stage	II	(T2)	Extension to cervix only
Stage	III	(T3)	Extension outside the uterus but confined to true pelvis
Stage	IV	(T4)	Extension beyond true pelvis or invading bladder or rectum

neoplastic cells shed from the ovary have free access to the peritoneal cavity, a considerably larger volume is encompassed by each stage than is common for other types of tumors. In addition, it should be noted that surgical findings are mandatory for determining the stage of an ovarian carcinoma.

Prior to surgery, distant metastases should be ruled out, but, in general, this mode of spread is uncommon. On the other hand, widespread intra-abdominal disease is difficult to detect prior to surgery, although computerized tomography should prove very useful for this purpose in the future. At present, contrast x rays of the gastrointestinal tract and lymphangiograms are more frequently used but have limited sensitivity. At the time of laparotomy, the surgeon must describe gross extent and volume of disease, including presence or absence of disease in lymph nodes and mesentery and the assumed completeness of resection as a guide for future management.

Head and Neck Cancer. Head and neck cancer is a grouping of several different types of tumors, each of which has its own rules for staging.[2] In general, they are based on size of disease when this can be easily measured (as in the oral cavity) or on areas of involvement (as in the larynx). Tables 3–9A, B and C provide precise staging rules.

Table 3–8. Staging of Ovarian Carcinoma[2]

OVARY			
Stage	I	(T1)	Growth limited to ovaries
	IA	(T1a)	Limited to one ovary, no ascites
		(T1ai)	Capsule intact
		(T1aii)	Capsule ruptured, or tumor on external surface, or both
	IB	(T1b)	Limited to both ovaries, no ascites
		(T1bi)	Capsule intact
		(T1bii)	Capsule ruptured, or tumor on external surface, or both
	IC	(T1c)	Either IA or IB with ascites
Stage	II	(T2)	Growth involving one or both ovaries with pelvic extension only
	IIA	(T2a)	Extension to uterus and/or tubes only
	IIB	(T2b)	Extension to other pelvic tissues
	IIC	(T2c)	Either IIA or IIB with ascites
Stage	III	(T3)	Spread outside pelvis or to retroperitoneal nodes or both
Stage	IV	(T4)	Spread to distant sites (pleural effusion must be confirmed histologically)

Table 3–9A. Staging of Oral Cavity Carcinoma[2]

TNM CLASSIFICATION

Primary tumor (T)

T0	No evidence of primary tumor
TIS	Carcinoma in situ
T1	Tumor 2 cm or less in greatest diameter
T2	Tumor greater than 2 cm but not greater than 4 cm in greatest diameter
T3	Tumor greater than 4 cm in greatest diameter
T4	Massive tumor greater than 4 cm in diameter with deep invasion to involve antrum, pterygoid muscles, root of tongue, or skin of neck

Nodal Involvement (N)

NX	Nodes cannot be assessed
N0	No clinically positive node
N1	Single clinically positive homolateral node less than 3 cm in diameter
N2	Single clinically positive homolateral node 3 to 6 cm in diameter or multiple clinically positive homolateral nodes, none over 6 cm in diameter
	N2a: Single clinically positive homolateral node, 3 to 6 cm in diameter
	N2b: Multiple clinically positive homolateral nodes, none over 6 cm in diameter
N3	Massive homolateral node(s), bilateral nodes, or contralateral node(s)
	N3a: Clinically positive homolateral node(s), over 6 cm in diameter
	N3b: Bilateral clinically positive nodes (in this situation, each side of the neck should be staged separately; that is, N3b: right, N2a: left, N1)
	N3c: Contralateral clinically positive node(s) only

Distant Metastasis (M)

MX	Not assessed
M0	No (known) distant metastasis
M1	Distant metastasis present
	Specify _____

Specify sites according to the following notations:

Pulmonary—PUL
Osseous—OSS
Hepatic—HEP
Brain—BRA
Lymph Nodes—LYM
Bone Marrow—MAR
Pleura—PLE
Skin—SKI
Eye—EYE
Other—OTH

Table 3–9A. (Cont'd)

STAGE GROUPING

Stage	I	T1 N0 M0
Stage	II	T2 N0 M0
Stage	III	T3 N0 M0
		T1 or T2 or T3, N1, M0
Stage	IV	T4, N0 or N1, M0
		Any T, N2 or N3, M0
		Any T, Any N, M1

The appropriate work-up of head and neck cancer varies, depending upon precise site of origin of the primary tumor. However, in all cases, careful inspection and *careful palpation* of the primary (when accessible) and potentially involved lymph node chains is vital. Lesions with indistinct borders can be clearly demonstrated by painting the involved region with toluidine blue which stains tumor but not normal surrounding epithelium. Inspection of virtually every head and neck site can be done by either mirrors or endoscopes. A soft tissue technique, lateral x ray of the neck may reveal a soft tissue mass in contrast to surrounding air passages as well as demonstrating cartilage destruction. Laryngograms, which outline laryngeal and hypopharyngeal structures by a radio-opaque dye, tomograms and computerized tomograms, all can be extremely helpful in defining extent of disease. Lesions of the nasopharynx require unique investigation because of their mode of spread. In general, tumors take the path of least resistance, which, in the case of nasopharyngeal tumors, is along the fascial planes which convey the tumor to the base of the skull near the jugular foramen and foramen lacerum. Thus, involvement of the base of skull is a relatively common finding in such disease, and x rays of the base of skull should routinely be done. Distant metastases from head and neck tumors occur uncommonly, and a chest x ray will detect most of them. However, undifferentiated tumors of the nasopharynx, in particular, and any markedly advanced tumor, in general, can spread to bone. In such cases a bone scan may well be worthwhile.

Brain. Staging of brain tumors is based on size and position of the lesion as indicated in Table 3–10.[2] As can be seen from the staging system, lymph node metastases from brain tumors do not occur and, in fact, distant metastases are extremely unusual.

Table 3–9B.   Staging of Laryngeal Carcinoma[2]

TNM CLASSIFICATION	
Primary Tumor (T)	
T0	No evidence of primary tumor
Supraglottis	
TIS	Carcinoma in situ
T1	Tumor confined to region of origin with normal mobility of vocal cords
T2	Tumor involving adjacent supraglottic site(s) or glottis without fixation of vocal cords
T3	Tumor limited to larynx with fixation and/or extension to involve postcricoid area, medial wall of pyriform sinus, or pre-epiglottic space
T4	Massive tumor extending beyond the larynx to involve oropharynx, soft tissues of neck, or destruction of thyroid cartilage
Glottis	
TIS	Carcinoma in situ
T1	Tumor confined to vocal cord(s) with normal mobility (including involvement of anterior or posterior commissures)
T2	Supraglottic and/or subglottic extension of tumor with normal or impaired cord mobility
T3	Tumor confined to the larynx with cord fixation
T4	Massive tumor with thyroid cartilage destruction and/or extension beyond the confines of the larynx
Subglottis	
TIS	Carcinoma in situ
T1	Tumor confined to the subglottic region
T2	Tumor extension to vocal cords with normal or impaired cord mobility
T3	Tumor confined to larynx with cord fixation
T4	Massive tumor with cartilage destruction or extension beyond the confines of the larynx, or both
Nodal Involvement (N)	
N0	No clinically positive node
N1	Single clinically positive homolateral node less than 3 cm in diameter
N2	Single clinically positive homolateral node 3 to 6 cm in diameter or multiple clinically positive homolateral nodes, none over 6 cm in diameter

Table 3–9B.   (Cont'd)

	N2a	Single clinically positive homolateral node, 3 to 6 cm in diameter
	N2b	Multiple clinically positive homolateral nodes, none over 6 cm in diameter
N3		Massive homolateral node(s), bilateral nodes, or contralateral node(s)
	N3a	Clinically positive homolateral node(s), over 6 cm in diameter
	N3b	Bilateral clinically positive nodes (in this situation, each side of the neck should be staged separately; that is N3b: right, N2a: left, N1)
	N3c	Contralateral clinically positive node(s) only

Distant Metastasis (M)
MX   Not assessed
M0   No (known) distant metastasis
M1   Distant metastasis present
           Specify _____
Specify sites according to the following notations:
            Pulmonary—PUL
            Osseous—OSS
            Hepatic—HEP
            Brain—BRA
        Lymph Nodes—LYM
        Bone Marrow—MAR
            Pleura—PLE
            Skin—SKI
            Eye—EYE
            Other—OTH

STAGE GROUPING
Stage   I   T1 N0 M0
Stage   II   T2 N0 M0
Stage   III   T3 N0 M0
                T1 or T2 or T3, N1, M0
Stage   IV   T4, N0 or N1, M0
                Any T, N2 or N3, M0
                Any T, Any N, M1

Table 3–9C.   Staging of Pharyngeal Carcinoma[2]

TNM CLASSIFICATION

Primary Tumor (T)

T0	No evidence of primary tumor

Nasopharynx

TIS	Carcinoma in situ
T1	Tumor confined to one site of nasopharynx or no tumor visible (positive biopsy only)
T2	Tumor involving two sites (both posterosuperior and lateral walls)
T3	Extension of tumor into nasal cavity or oropharynx
T4	Tumor invasion of skull or cranial nerve involvement, or both

Oropharynx

TIS	Carcinoma in situ
T1	Tumor 2 cm or less in greatest diameter
T2	Tumor greater than 2 cm, but not greater than 4 cm in greatest diameter
T3	Tumor greater than 4 cm in greatest diameter
T4	Massive tumor greater than 4 cm in diameter with invasion of bone, soft tissues of neck, or root (deep musculature) of tongue

Hypopharynx

TIS	Carcinoma in situ
T1	Tumor confined to the site of origin
T2	Extension of tumor to adjacent region or site without fixation of hemilarynx
T3	Extension of tumor to adjacent region or site with fixation of hemilarynx
T4	Massive tumor invading bone or soft tissues of neck

Nodal Involvement (N)

NX	Nodes cannot be assessed
N0	No clinically positive node
N1	Single clinically positive homolateral node less than 3 cm in diameter
N2	Single clinically positive homolateral node 3 to 6 cm in diameter or multiple clinically positive homolateral node, none over 6 cm in diameter
N2a	Single clinically positive homolateral node, 3 to 6 cm in diameter
N2b	Multiple clinically positive homolateral nodes, none over 6 cm in diameter
N3	Massive homolateral node(s), bilateral nodes or contralateral node(s)
N3a	Clinically positive homolateral node(s), over 6 cm in diameter
N3b	Bilateral clinically positive nodes (in this situation, each side of the neck should be staged separately: that is, N3b; right, N2a; left N1)
N3c	Contralateral clinically positive node(s) only

Distant Metastasis (M)

MX	Not assessed
M0	No (known) distant metastasis
M1	Distant metastasis present
	Specify _____

Table 3–9C.   (Cont'd)

Specify sites according to the following notations:
Pulmonary—PUL
Osseous—OSS
Hepatic—HEP
Brain—BRA
Lymph Nodes—LYM
Bone Marrow—MAR
Pleura—PLE
Skin—SKI
Eye—EYE
Other—OTH

Table 3–10.   Staging of Brain Tumors[2]

TNM CLASSIFICATION
Primary Tumor (T)
Supratentorial Tumor:
T1   Greatest diameter is less than 5 cm; confined to one side
T2   Greatest diameter is more than 5 cm; confined to one side
T3   Greatest diameter may be less than 5 cm; invades or encroaches upon the ventricular system
T4   Crosses the midline, invades the opposite hemisphere, or extends infratentorially
Infratentorial Tumor:
T1   Greatest diameter is less than 3 cm; confined to one side
T2   Greatest diameter is more than 3 cm; confined to one side
T3   Greatest diameter may be less than 3 cm; invades or encroaches upon the ventricular system
T4   Crosses the midline, invades the opposite hemisphere, or extends supratentorially
Node Involvement (N)—Does not apply to this site
Distant Metastasis (M)
MX   Not assessed
M0   No (known) distant metastasis
M1   Distant metastasis present
Specify _____
Specify sites according to the following notations:
Subarachnoid Space—CSF
Pulmonary—PUL
Lymph Nodes—LYM
Osseous—OSS
Hepatic—HEP
Bone Marrow—MAR
Other—OTH

Work-up of brain tumors basically seeks to define the location and extent of tumor, thereby permitting the neurosurgeon to evaluate the feasibility of resection and, if possible, the appropriate approach. Conventional skull x rays, radioisotopic brain scans, cerebral angiograms and computerized tomograms all contribute such information. Work-up for distant metastatic disease is virtually unnecessary in the case of primary brain tumors; however, a thorough review of body systems needs to be done to exclude the possibility that cerebral lesions are metastases from other sites.

References

1. Podolsky, D.K., et al.: A Cancer-Associated Galactosyltransferase Isoenzyme. N. Engl. J. Med. 299:703–705, 1978.
2. Manual For Staging of Cancer 1977, Chicago, American Joint Committee for Cancer Staging and End-Results Reporting, 1977.
3. Astler, V.B., and Coller, F.A.: The Prognostic Significance of Direct Extension of Carcinoma of the Colon and Rectum. Ann. Surg. 139:846–852, 1954.

4

THE ONCOLOGIST

The oncologist accepts responsibility for determining and supervising appropriate anticancer therapy. Although type and extent of disease may suggest several acceptable choices of treatment, only one plan can be recommended. This compels the oncologist to wear several hats.

To begin with, the oncologist must be an expert in neoplastic disease, thoroughly schooled in the biologic behavior of tumors. Every type of tumor has an inherent nature which should be exploited by the treatment plan. Also, the oncologist must be a detective using clues in the patient's history and physical examination, or characteristic patterns of tumor behavior seen in similar patients, to uncover the extent of disease. Furthermore, medicine is an art, as well as a science; judgment and experience must complement factual knowledge. In oncology, as in other medical subspecialties, optimal management does not result simply by following directions in a cookbook of therapy. Thus, the oncologist must also be an analyst and tactician, processing information about potential gains and complications of various forms of management and applying it to the individual patient.

In addition, medicine cannot be practiced in a vacuum. Each patient is unique, with specific fears and needs that can influence the selection of therapy. Some patients categorically refuse to consider having surgery or radiotherapy or chemotherapy; some refuse all therapy. At times, they associate their problem with those of a friend or relative who fared poorly after a particular form of management. At other times they are influenced by the media, by reports of unnecessary surgery, by fictional monsters created by radiation, or by futile efforts of chemotherapy to save the beautiful young heroine of a sad, romantic motion picture. Thus, the oncologist must be a judge, knowing when alternative therapy, in keeping with the patient's preferences is reasonable, and when patients' wishes would substantially impair their chances of having a successful outcome. Of course, the oncologist must also recognize when therapy is unlikely to benefit the patient. Patients should not be denied hope, but it is unconscionable to administer therapy for its *placebo* value when therapy often includes unpleasant side effects and difficult-to-manage complications.

Last, although available methods clearly are inadequate to deal with all situations satisfactorily, and new methods need to be devised to improve survival, until such methods are proven in controlled experimental trials, they should not be offered to the occasional patient. The title of *Oncologist* is *NOT* a license to perform uncontrolled experiments. The "Oncologist" who treats patients by copying the latest "soup-de-jour" being investigated by a research center, is mentioned solely to be condemned. If a patient wishes to receive experimental therapy, with its greater attendant potential for success *and* greater potential risk of failure and complications, he or she should receive such therapy as part of a study group, both to benefit subsequent patients by the knowledge to be gained from the study and to avail him or herself of the medical resources of the group. When experimental therapy consists of a series of anecdotal experiences, neither medical science nor particular patients treated are likely to benefit greatly.

The oncologist has many responsibilities, solving puzzles by available methods, trying to maximize gains and minimize risks. The purpose of this chapter is to discuss the role the oncologist plays and, in particular, to examine his or her training, specific expertise, and responsiblity to the referring physician.

Who is the Oncologist? Thus far the title "Oncologist" has been used to designate any physician who specializes in the treatment of neoplastic disease; however, in reality, there are several different kinds of oncologists. There are medical oncologists, radiation oncologists, and surgical oncologists, with the latter category including head and neck surgical oncologists and gynecologic oncologists. Consequently, the referring physician initially must decide which type of oncologist (or types of oncologists) to consult.

For many years, because of the tradition of oncologic management by surgery in the United States, the surgeon has been regarded as the primary decision maker in cancer therapy. This differs from the situation in Europe where radiotherapy has played a dominant role and the radiotherapist is considered the cancer doctor. In fact, neither solution is totally adequate. General surgery training programs rarely include formal training in radiation oncology or medical oncology. Most surgeons' "expertise" in these areas is picked up on the job, frequently from other surgeons. The general radiologist or hematologist, who practices oncology part-time, probably is no better off, even though he or she received some surgical training in medical school and may have done an internship which included surgical training. While current training in all oncologic subspecialties surely is more comprehensive than in the past, cancer therapy is so complex that no individual can be expert in surgical therapy, radiotherapy *and* chemotherapy. It can therefore be asked "Is any subspecialty group entitled to consider itself 'The Oncologists'?" We think not. And yet, it is only the fortunate patient who is seen by all three subspecialists prior to therapy. Even today, although it has become accepted policy for third party carriers (Insurance Companies) to accept or demand a second opinion prior to a surgical procedure, seldom is there similar pressure for consultation with a medical or radiation oncologist prior to a surgical oncologic procedure.

And, what prospect is there of an omniscient oncologist in the future? DeVita[1] asks "Will systemic treatment become so simple that all treatment will be given by surgeons? . . . . Will much of cancer surgery be replaced by high linear-energy transfer particulate radiotherapy with computerized, precise delivery, coupled with systemic treatment, that could, after all, be given by radiotherapists? . . . . Will medical oncologists treat everyone after only a diagnostic biopsy by a general surgeon or even the medical oncologist?" Not likely. Neoplastic cells and normal cells appear to be too similar to permit any one modality always to be successful by itself. On the other hand, multidisciplinary attacks, utilizing specific expertise of several types of oncologists provides a logical approach.

The Current Oncologist. In light of previous questions, it is appropriate to review the training required of various oncologic subspecialists to aid physicians in requesting consultation.

Surgical Oncology. Surgical oncologists, other than gynecologic oncologists, are trained basically as general surgeons. Subsequently, they specialize in cancer surgery but at present there are no specialty boards to attest to their competence. Surgeons can express interest in the field by becoming members of the Society of Surgical Oncology,

Inc. (formerly the James Ewing Society), or in one of the subspecialty societies such as the Society of Head and Neck Surgeons, or the American Society for Head and Neck Surgery. Moreover, they are eligible for membership in such multidisciplinary groups as the American Radium Society, Inc., and the American Society of Clinical Oncology, Inc. Gynecologic oncologists must be Diplomates of the American Board of Obstetrics and Gynecology, and must have completed a 2-year program in gynecologic oncology (or its equivalent) to be eligible for board certification as an oncologist. The national organization of these physicians is the Society of Gynecologic Oncologists.

Radiation Oncology. Current requirements for board certification in therapeutic radiology include a minimum of 3 years of residency in a radiation oncology program. In addition to formal instruction in the mechanics of radiation therapy, such training must include a fundamental background in cancer biology and pathology as well as surgical and medical oncology. Exposure to statistical analysis and research also is required. In addition, a fourth post-graduate study year in radiation oncology or in a related field is required to broaden expertise. The American Society of Therapeutic Radiologists is the national organization of radiation oncology and many therapeutic radiologists also belong to multimodality groups, such as the American Radium Society and the American Society of Clinical Oncology, Inc.

Medical Oncology. Training requirements for medical oncology recently have been clarified.[2] Practitioners must first be certified in general internal medicine and then participate in training programs which are similar to those operational in radiation oncology, requiring working knowledge of cancer biology, pathology, statistics, surgery and radiotherapy while acquiring expertise in chemotherapy. The American Society of Clinical Oncology, Inc., serves as the national organization of medical oncology, and many chemotherapists belong to other oncologic societies.

The Consult. Whatever the subspecialty of the oncology consultant, his task is to devise a rational strategy for treatment of the patient. From the previous discussions it should be clear that in any given case there may be more than one effective plan to be considered. If the likelihood of cure is equivalent, secondary factors such as morbidity of treatment, length of time of treatment, necessity of hospitalization for treatment, and so forth, can and should be considered both by the patient and referring physician. Information necessary for such decisions should be clearly presented in the oncologist's consultation.

We believe that every consultation should, at a minimum, contain (1) *pertinent* recapitulation of the patient's history, physical examination and laboratory data to date; (2) an overall assessment of the problem, including any additional studies that are necessary prior to recommendation for or against treatment; (3) description of the extent of disease, i.e., staging (see Chap. 3); (4) definition of intention of treatment, i.e., cure, palliation, prophylaxis (Chap. 14); (5) proposed method of treatment, and (6) likely benefits and risks of treatment. In some cases a number of methods of treatment should be discussed, and if the proposed treatment is either uncommon or new, literature references should be provided. When these specific points are considered, the actual value of a consult may be judged. Note the difference between the following hypothetical examples.

The Inadequate Consult. The patient is a 53-year-old female, gravida 3, para 3003, last menstrual period 3 years ago, who came to the emergency room last Tuesday complaining of vaginal bleeding. Several weeks ago, she first experienced vaginal bleeding which recurred 4 times over the past 4 weeks and prompted her to seek medical advice. She has had many negative PAP smears in the past and, aside from gallstone removal 10 years ago, was in good health.

On admission to the hospital she was not bleeding, but upon examination, a lesion of the cervix was evident. Biopsy subsequently revealed it to be carcinoma. Work-up thus far shows:

Bloods: Hct 27, Hgb 9.2, WBC 5.8, platelets 250,000
Chemistries: Sodium 140, potassium 4.6, chloride 98, CO_2 30, urea nitrogen 10,
             creatinine 0.6, glucose 100, SGOT 40, SGPT 45, LDH 100, CPK 250
X rays: Chest—normal, IVP—normal, GI series—normal
Other: Sigmoidoscopy—normal to 25 cm

This patient should be treated by cobalt irradiation and intracavitary radium. Please transfer to radiation therapy service.

The Adequate Consult. The patient is a 53-year-old white female, with biopsy proven squamous cell carcinoma of the cervix who presented with a 2-month history of vaginal bleeding. Physical examination, upon admission, revealed an exophytic lesion occupying the left side of the cervical face only. Punch biopsy of the lesion was reported as moderately differentiated squamous cell carcinoma.

The patient has no known etiologic risk factors. She never has had pelvic surgery or pelvic radiotherapy, and other than her cervical disease, has no significant medical history.

On physical examination today, the patient is in good general condition without adenopathy or hepatomegaly. Pelvic examination reveals a friable, exophytic, 2 cm lesion occupying the left hemicervix, The vagina, parametria and rectovaginal septum are free of disease.

Work-up including blood count, chemistries, chest x ray and IVP is significant only for anemia (Hgb 9.2).

In summary, the patient has localized stage IB disease. It is recommended that she receive radiotherapy with the intention of treatment being cure of disease. The primary tumor should be treated by intracavitary radiotherapy (which will require placement under general anesthesia and confine the patient to the hospital for two stays of 3 to 4 days each). The risk of pelvic lymph node metastases is approximately 15% and external beam radiotherapy should be given to the nodes at risk (over a 5-week period of daily treatment which can be given on an outpatient basis). Prior to therapy the patient should be transfused to a hemoglobin of at least 13.5.

Therapy as outlined should provide a 75 to 80% probability of cure of disease with less than a 5% risk of complications.

Alternative surgical therapy can be considered and consultation with the Gynecologic Oncology Service is advised.

Clinical Trials. Despite the oncologist's experience and all the accumulated information used to predict the efficacy of various regimens for a specific tumor, the fact exists that optimal treatment for a particular situation, frequently is not known. In such cases, the oncologist may advise one regimen that appears to be as good as any other, or he or she may offer the patient entry into an experimental trial, designed to determine the better regimen.

Experimental trials are of two basic types: *retrospective* (historical) and *prospective* (randomized) trials.

Retrospective studies are so named because they compare treatment regimens that were given in the past. Comparisons of results of the same type of treatment during two different time periods, or of different treatments occurring during different time periods, exemplify historical analyses.

Occasionally, a treatment is discovered that has considerable promise. Naturally, physicians want to use the method for their patients and, in fact, withholding the new treatment might be considered unethical. Yet, because the method is new and largely untried, the precise degree of benefit will be unknown. Retrospective studies, comparing results of the new treatment to the results of methods formerly used to treat the same disease, may be the only way of demonstrating its value.

Nobody, for example, would seriously consider withholding penicillin from some patients who have pneumococcal pneumonia while giving it to others, solely to prove that the drug is effective.

Unfortunately, the effect of most medical regimens is less dramatic and the manner in which patients are selected to receive therapy, rather than the treatment itself, can lead to erroneous conclusions. For example, Jaffe et al.[3] reported that between 1972 and 1974, adjuvant chemotherapy, given after operation or radiation for osteogenic sarcomas *significantly* reduced the incidence of subsequent pulmonary metastases, when compared to their incidence in patients treated without chemotherapy between 1950 and 1972.

As evidence that factors other than chemotherapy could have played only a minor role in reducing the incidence of metastases, the authors demonstrated similar survival rates during the entire "historical control" period, implying that any change must be the result of the new treatment. By itself, the evidence seems clear. However, Taylor et al.[4] have analyzed their results in patients having osteogenic sarcomas, treated without chemotherapy from 1963 to 1974, and found a progressive *increase* in survival during this period, even though treatment remained the same. In fact, they note that their most recent results without chemotherapy are similar to those of other authors advocating chemotherapy. Thus, retrospective studies often fail to prove their point convincingly.

To avoid ambiguous results, *prospective randomized* trials have been developed. In such studies, two or more different treatment regimens which appear to be equally effective are formalized so that the minute details of each regimen can be applied uniformly to any patient. Then, any patient who wishes to participate in the study randomly is assigned to one of the regimens. In this manner, any patient factor(s) which might influence outcome, are evenly distributed throughout treatment groups, and their effects should cancel out. Unfortunately, this scheme demands that (1) patients be willing to accept any one of the treatment regimens, (2) details of each regimen be followed meticulously, (3) investigators not be biased in data collection, and (4) large numbers of patients be available for study, since the number of patients who can receive any one form of treatment is inversely proportional to the number of treatment options. Despite these substantial difficulties, whenever feasible, prospective studies are preferable to retrospective studies because their conclusions are more reliable.

Data Evaluation. Whether obtained from prospective or retrospective analyses, survival data should be presented in a manner which permits the reader to comprehend its meaning easily. In general, such data are displayed in tabular or graphic form, depicting "5-year survival." However, 5-year survival can be calculated in several different ways and the unwary reader can be led to an erroneous conclusion.

Crude 5-year survival rates provide the most basic data. Only the number of patients who were treated 5 or more years ago are considered. The rate is determined by the ratio of the number alive at 5 years to the total number treated. Unfortunately, this method ignores information available from patients who were treated less than 5 years ago and does not consider death from other causes.

Actuarial or life-table 5-year survival rates utilize data from all patients as long as some patients have been followed for 5 years. In addition, the method compensates for patients who are lost to follow-up. While the method does provide more information than crude rates, one must carefully examine *how many* patients have actually been followed for 5 years and *how much* of the analysis is projected from lesser follow-up.

Adjusted 5-year survival rates are similar to actuarial rates except that an adjustment compensates for the number of deaths that were not related to cancer.

Relative survival rates provide the same information; however, in the former method, the precise number of deaths unrelated to cancer must be known while in the latter method it need not. Relative rates adjust the survival of each member of the study group by a factor determined from the survival of "normal" persons of the same age, sex and race throughout the nation.

For the reader who would like to learn the mechanics of each of these types of analysis, a clear, concise explanation can be found in the *Manual for Staging of Cancer.*[5]

Follow-up. Although the oncologist's responsibility primarily occurs prior to and during therapy, the oncologist must also provide follow-up care after treatment. Four basic factors demand that the cancer victim, particularly if he or she is likely to be cured, receive follow-up care and the oncologist must be prepared to provide this care. *First*, some unfortunate individuals are predisposed to multiple tumors. At least some cancer victims suffer a higher than average chance of developing a subsequent tumor. A patient who is found to have a head and neck tumor has a 10 to 15% risk of having or developing another tumor within the upper aerodigestive tract alone. *Second*, the biologic behavior of the treated tumor must be used as a rational guide of the frequency and type of follow-up. Breast cancers not uncommonly recur beyond 5 years after treatment so that follow-up must continue for many years. In contrast, head and neck cancers recur rapidly, and, therefore, follow-up should be spaced at short intervals. In any case, the type and number of procedures that should be done at each follow-up visit, must be based on natural history of disease. *Third*, several types of tumors display unique behavior during follow-up. For example, embryonal carcinomas of the testis, which have metastasized to lungs and are treated by chemotherapy, may regress initially but then fail to disappear. Although one *might* assume that the tumor had become chemoresistant, it is well established that residual lesions not infrequently are benign teratomas requiring surgical excision. *Fourth*, iatrogenic reactions and complications secondary to treatment must be sought and detected as early as possible to facilitate successful management.

References

1. DeVita, V.T., Jr.: The Evolution of Therapeutic Research in Cancer. N. Engl. J. Med. *298*:907–910, 1978.
2. The Subspecialty of Oncology, Guidelines of the American Board of Internal Medicine. Semin. Oncol. *4*:i–v, 1977.
3. Jaffe, N., *et al.*: Adjuvant Methotrexate and Citrovorum-Factor Treatment of Osteogenic Sarcoma. N. Engl. J. Med. *291*:994–1000, 1974.
4. Taylor, W.F., *et al.*: Trends and Variability in Survival from Osteosarcoma. Mayo Clin. Proc. *53*:695–700, 1978.
5. Manual for Staging of Cancer 1977, Chicago, American Joint Committee for Cancer Staging and End-Results Reporting, 1977.

THE RATIONALE

Cellular Level

5

EFFECT OF CELL TYPE

Despite the immense variation in appearance and behavior of multicellular life, all life begins as a single cell. This cell grows and divides, eventually producing a unique organism whose nature largely is determined by the genetic composition of its progenitor cell.

Tumors arise in the same fashion and, in consequence, the characteristics of any lesion basically can be attributed to its cell of origin. For this reason, the next four chapters examine non-surgical oncology at the cellular level. In particular, this chapter discusses the effect of cell type.

The Aim of Therapy. Odd as it may seem, cancer cells need not be killed during treatment for a beneficial effect to occur. Instead nonsurgical therapeutic methods make cells of cancers unable to reproduce. When this has been accomplished, the cancer will be unable to grow, spread into surrounding tissues or metastasize to distant sites. Moreover, when sterile cancer cells die, the cancer will shrink, and if all cells in the cancer are sterilized by treatment, the growth will, in time, vanish. Thus, non-surgical therapeutic techniques aim to destroy the *reproductive potential* of cancer cells and, because this is true, a great deal of effort has been spent in studying how chemotherapeutic agents and ionizing radiations affect reproductive potential.

Ionizing Radiation. Despite considerable effort, no conclusive evidence firmly establishes exactly how radiation damages cellular reproductive potential. However, it seems clear that as dose * increases,

* Radiation dose is measured by the amount of radiant energy absorbed in tissue, and expressed in the unit "rad." One rad signifies absorption of 100 ergs per gram of irradiated tissue. Common radiotherapeutic regimens deliver approximately 200 rad per day.

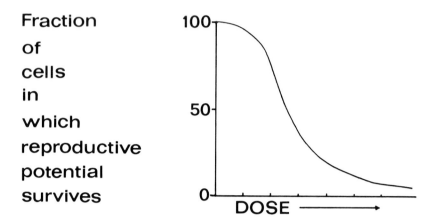

Fraction of cells in which reproductive potential survives

Fig. 5–1. *Survival of reproductive potential in a population of human cells irradiated with increasing doses of the radiations most commonly used in radiation therapy (x rays, gamma rays and electrons). Through low dose ranges few cells are sterilized. A point is reached at which the curve bends and a steep slope follows. From this point on, large fractions of the population are made sterile by incremental doses which, at low dose levels, would sterilize few.*

the probability that cellular reproductive potential will be irrevocably lost also increases. When common types of radiations are tested, a distinctive dose-effect pattern emerges that applies to *nearly* all human cells (Fig. 5–1).

The pattern suggests that, in low dose ranges, few cells are sufficiently damaged to be sterilized. A dose level is reached, however, at which the dose-effect curve bends sharply and a steep slope follows. Evidently, at that point, much of the population becomes quite vulnerable to sterilization by added radiation. No one is certain what happens in cells to produce this change, but a common hypothesis states that reproductive potential is lost only when a number of sites (or targets) in cells have been destroyed.

In this manner, the mechanisms responsible for reproductive potential can be seen to be analogous in design to backup systems in complex machinery. Several of such systems can fail before the machine becomes inoperative, because each system, by itself, assures function.

Through low dose ranges, the likelihood of destroying all cellular sites assuring reproductive potential is small and few cells are sterilized. But, within these same dose ranges, some sites are destroyed, and, as dose gets higher, greater numbers are destroyed. Eventually the bulk of the population will have only one site remaining undestroyed. Additional radiation now has a good chance of destroying that site in many cells, making them sterile. A sudden sharp decrease in the proliferative fraction occurs, represented by the sudden change in the slope of the dose-effect curve. This point of inflection can be viewed as a kind of "threshold dose" separating a *low* probability of loss of reproductive potential from a high probability of loss of reproductive potential.

Cell Type. The point or dose at which the threshold occurs differs among various cell types. It would be useful in therapy, if cancer cells had a low threshold and normal cells a high one. Differences, even if small, might be exploitable. Unfortunately, although the value differs among cell types, little difference exists between those of cancers and *the normal tissues from which they were derived*. Moreover, the threshold is not always lower for cancer than for normal tissues; sometimes cancers' thresholds are lower, sometimes higher.

Considerable effort has been expended trying to learn how thresholds might be altered. If thresholds could be raised or lowered—it might be possible to lower that of the cancer cell population either without moving that of normal tissues at all, or lowering that of normal tissue less than that of cancers. If that could be done, certain doses of radiation might fall *above* the threshold of cancers—and sterilize many of its cells—but *below* that of normal tissue and sterilize relatively fewer of its cells. Efforts are complicated by the lack of knowledge about exactly what is injured in cells when they become sterile. Nevertheless, changes in threshold can be produced by changing oxygen tension, using highly charged radiations and altering the *rate* at which conventionally used radiations are delivered. Evidence also shows that chemicals added to cells can change the threshold either by making it greater—protectors, or making it smaller—sensitizers. Substantial interest exists in these methods and trials in animal models and clinical settings are now under way. All show promise but none yet can be applied generally. It will take time, but some, if not all, of these methods likely will find their way into standard practice in the not-too-distant future.

Radiosensitivity. So far the threshold of the dose-response curve has been discussed, but this is only one feature of the curve. A second is the steep slope following the threshold. Since in this dose range, cells are being sterilized, the *slope* of this segment of the curve represents another parameter—namely radiosensitivity. It indicates how effi-

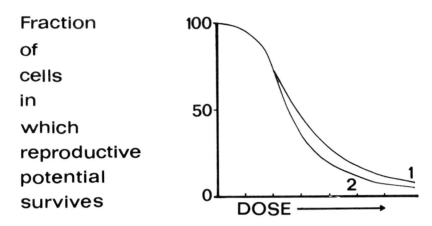

Fig. 5-2. *Two dose-response curves having the same threshold but different final slopes. Curves (1) and (2) have the same threshold; they bend sharply down at the same point. However, the subsequent slope is* steeper *in curve (2) than in (1).*

ciently radiation produces irrevocable loss of the function, reproduction (Fig. 5-2). Two populations of cells may have the same threshold but different response to irradiation thereafter. The portion of the dose-effect curve following the threshold describes the liability of cells to sustain irrevocable loss of reproductive capacity. In Figure 5-2, the cell population in curve (2) exhibits greater sensitivity to radiation than that of curve (1). The slope of that curve is *steeper* than that of curve (1). *Radiosensitivity* may be exploited to advantage in cancer therapy. If tumor cells are more sensitive than *normal* cells, then doses—in excess of the threshold dose—would sterilize more cancer cells than normal cells. Unfortunately, although substantial differences in radiosensitivity of various cell types exist, cancer cells usually are not very different from normal cells *of the same type* in this regard. For instance, leukemia, a neoplasm of bone marrow, is about as *radiosensitive* as bone marrow itself. But leukemia is quite radiosensitive compared to numerous normal tissues. Leukemic cells, sequestered in brain, will succumb to radiation doses not *expected* to produce much damage to brain. Similarly, lymphoma cells are quite radiosensitive and lesions in various more resistant normal tissues can be treated without producing much normal tissue change.

Differential sensitivity can work *against* the success of radiotherapy also. If a resistant tumor spreads to a sensitive region, normal tissue tolerance precludes effective radiation. Normal tissue would be destroyed before the dose would be high enough to sterilize the tumor.

Efforts have been directed to find means to change the slope of survival curves. Heavy particles used as radiations accomplish this; so do changes in radiation dose rate. Numerous drugs (true and false sensitizers) are also effective (Chap. 11). More time is needed before these methods can be adopted as common clinical tools; perhaps, in time, it will be possible for the oncologist to change sensitivity at will and greatly improve patient care.

Radioresponsiveness. It may already have come to mind that, if threshold radiation doses for cancer and normal tissues are similar, and if radiosensitivity of malignant and normal tissue of origin are also similar, how can anyone expect cancers and normal tissues to respond to radiation differently from each other? The reason is that threshold and sensitivity are qualities of cells, but *radioresponsiveness* is a quality of *masses* of cells, whether well-organized ones, like tissues or organs, or less well-organized ones, like cancers. Radiation causes cell loss and high doses cause large losses. Normal tissues and organs, under host homeostatic control, are prepared to deal with cell loss. In nearly all tissues and organs adjustment for cell loss is a natural, everyday occurrence. We are cut or scraped. The injured tissue responds, under homeostatic control, by supplying cells quickly. The cut heals, the scrape covers over. If we bleed, the hemopoietic system produces many new cells and normal levels are restored. An organ is irradiated. Many cells die. The organ responds by supplying new cells to take their place. But cancers are not under such control. When they lose many cells, they do not respond by producing many new ones to fill the deficit. They simply produce cells at or near their usual rate. Cell type greatly influences radioresponsiveness and in a way that can to some extent be predicted. *Radiation injury* primarily involves proliferative cells, as will be discussed in Chapter 7. But, tissues and organs normally respond to the loss of *non-proliferative* functional cells. The homeostatic mechanism seems to recognize loss of functional cells and responds to replace *depressed function*. Normal tissues with a naturally high loss of functional cells, blood and mucosal linings, for example, respond to irradiation quickly. The radiation produced loss of proliferative cells *and* the natural loss of functional cells quickly combine to cause a drop in function. Homeostatic controls recognize this and react by bringing about quick repopulation.

Normal tissue with naturally low loss of functional cells, muscle and nerve, for example, do not respond to irradiation quickly. No loss of function is immediately obvious and little or no repopulation occurs.

Clinical Aspects. While the previous discussion of radiosensitivity describes changes in tumor cell population secondary to treatment in precise terms, it fails to provide an indication of which tumors are sufficiently sensitive to be commonly treated by radiotherapy. In part this seeming paradox can be explained by noting that factors other than the inherent sensitivity of the basic cell type of a tumor alter tumor response to treatment, as will be described in subsequent chapters. In addition, the efficacy of any form of management cannot fairly be evaluated in a vacuum; it must be compared to the results that are possible with other methods. Nevertheless, several types of cancers respond sufficiently well to be treated by radiation with the expectation of cure of disease.

Testicular Seminoma. Seminomas are the most common type of testicular neoplasm, most victims being between 20 and 45 years old when affected. Spread of disease predominantly occurs via the lymphatic system, many patients remaining free of hematogenous metastases despite gross para-aortic nodal involvement. Biopsy of a suspected testis is contraindicated and radical orchiectomy must be done to establish the diagnosis and as a first step in therapy. Once accomplished, radiation therapy should be employed for all remaining lymphatic disease including a margin of tissue containing the next chain of draining lymphatics which appears to be uninvolved (Chap. 10). Modest doses of radiation uniformly suffice.[1,2] Doses approximating one-half that required for most other types of tumors produce cure of disease in 90% of cases.

Hodgkin's Disease. Hodgkin's disease is a lymphoma characterized by the presence of a specific type of cell—the so-called Reed-Sternberg cell. Most affected patients are in their late teens or early adulthood although a second cluster of patients is in their 50s. Four histopathological variants are recognized: lymphocyte predominance, nodular sclerosing, mixed cell, and lymphocyte depletion. Although the disease is more likely to be aggressive and to be detected in an advanced stage with lymphocyte depletion or mixed cellular types of disease than with nodular sclerosing or lymphocyte predominance, no difference in radioresponsiveness occurs among subtypes.

Hodgkin's disease probably is the paradigm of a radiocurable tumor. The careful studies and tested methods of Kaplan[3,4] and his associates, which demonstrated that the disease spreads in a predictable, contiguous fashion, provide clear guidance in the curative treatment of

Hodgkin's lymphoma by sophisticated radiotherapy. At present, cure can be expected in 80 to 90% of Stage I and Stage II patients.

Non-Hodgkin's Lymphoma. Unlike that of Hodgkin's disease, the spread of non-Hodgkin's lymphoma is unpredictable. Consequently, it most frequently must be treated by systemic means as will shortly be described. However, the tumor itself is radiosensitive and when discovered in a localized state, clearly is radiocurable[5,6] with doses only slightly greater than those necessary for Hodgkin's disease.

Epithelial Cancers. Epithelial cancers account for the majority of tumors. And it is with these lesions, in particular, skin, breast, prostate, cervix, and head and neck tumors, that radiotherapy frequently demonstrates its efficacy, as was described in Chapter 2. In addition, several other less common epithelial neoplasms, such as bladder[7,8] and esophageal[9] cancers are radiocurable in their earlier stages. Unfortunately, the epithelial tumors require greater doses than do the lymphomas, doses that may approach tissue tolerance of adjacent normal organs.

Non-Epithelial Tumors. As a group, non-epithelial tumors, including melanomas and brain tumors are the least responsive general class of neoplasms. Although there are some notable exceptions, such as medulloblastomas, lesion for lesion, dose for dose, less response should be expected from these tumors than from those already discussed. However, this should not be interpreted to mean that they are not radiotreatable. In the proper circumstances, radiotherapy can be the treatment of choice[10-14] but may require high doses or uncommon treatment schedules.

Palliative Irradiation. Independent of the type of tumor, *most* tumors are sufficiently sensitive to radiation that at least some regression of disease can be expected in most cases. Often shrinkage will occur with relatively low doses. Consequently, patients who are beyond a reasonable expectation of achieving cure of their disease, can be offered low dose (to avoid side effects) palliation of distressing symptoms by radiotherapy. In such cases the small degree of regression produced substantially decreases the patient's discomfort and improves the quality of survival.

Chemotherapy. Chemotherapy literally means treatment by chemicals. In current usage, however, the term implies the beneficial use of drugs for the treatment of patients who have a malignancy. Such drugs are administered in a variety of ways: oral, intramuscular, intravenous, and intra-arterial. In general, they circulate throughout the body and there are few sites in which they are not active (Chap. 11). Occasionally they are used in a regionalized fashion (similar to radiotherapy), restricted to limited sites. This can be done by infusion techniques, where the drug is delivered directly to the tumor, or perfusion techniques, where the drug is recirculated through an isolated region. Most of these drugs act to disrupt cellular biosynthesis and a description of the various mechanisms of action is included in Chapter 7. Unfortunately, these drugs also act to poison normal cells. If the effect against tumor cells is greater than the effect against normal cells, the drug has clinical value. However, even in such cases, the therapeutic ratio is so small that these drugs must be considered highly toxic and prescribed with caution.

In addition to cytotoxic drugs, chemotherapy includes treatment of tumors by hormonal manipulation. This type of therapy is based on the expectation that some characteristics of the parent tissue were retained by the tumor. If the parent organ normally responds to hormonal stimuli, such as is the case in breast, endometrium and prostate, there is a reasonable expectation that tumors derived from these organs may respond to hormonal control. Such hormonal manipulation is without cytotoxic effect, and adverse reactions to these agents therefore are physiologic, usually of a mild nature and considerably less common than with cytotoxic chemotherapeutic agents because of the differences between cytotoxic and hormonal therapy. Treatment by hormonal means will be described in Chapter 6.

Sensitivity to Chemotherapy. Sensitivity of tumors to chemotherapy varies considerably. In some cases, marked sensitivity exists and treatment produces control of disease. In others, sensitivity is moderate and only palliation of distressing symptoms can be obtained. In some, currently available drugs do not produce any clinical benefit.

The reader undoubtedly understands the intended meaning of "sensitivity to chemotherapy." In essence, it implies more frequent control or regression of disease from a lesser absorbed dose of drug than occurs with other cancers from larger drug doses. However, this is difficult to demonstrate. Unlike radiotherapy, wherein doses are prescribed in terms of precisely calibrated amounts of absorbed energy, chemotherapy doses are measured by the weight of drug given. Because of possible routes of administration, the variation in absorption, possible enzymatic degradation and deficiencies of transport of drug to the tumor (Chap. 11), quantitation of dose absorbed by the tumor is only approximate. In addition, varying size of patients affects dilution of drug. Prescription of doses based on a milligram of drug per kilogram of body weight or milligram of drug per square meter of body surface area ameliorates some of the problem. Even so, the term *chemotherapy* encompasses so wide a variety of drugs, all of which have slightly different actions, indications and toxicities that the effect of a milligram of one drug may have no relation to a milligram of another.

A second difficulty in describing sensitivity to chemotherapy reflects the narrow therapeutic range of most cytotoxic drugs in man. Because most drugs show little, if any, therapeutic benefit until doses which come quite close to toxicity are reached, there is a narrow dose range over which most drugs are prescribed. Thus, most tumors are described as being sensitive or insensitive to a particular drug (given in conventional dosage) rather than being described as sensitive to a particular dose of a drug. There is no question, however, that a relationship between drug dosage and tumor response does exist.

Last, sensitivity has to be described in relation to a specific regimen. A tumor which is totally insensitive to one drug can be extremely sensitive to another. When potent *combinations of drugs* are used to produce complete regression of disease, sensitivity is obviously difficult to define.

Thus, "sensitivity to chemotherapy" is an elusive concept to define precisely. Nonetheless, the concept has great clinical relevance and consequently some basic guidelines are therefore presented.

Effect of Cell Type on Chemotherapy. As might be expected, tumor cell type influences treatment by chemotherapy. The wide variation in sensitivity of disease to chemotherapy is, in fact, somewhat predictable on the basis of cell type. This is not to say that a tumor which is likely to be highly chemosensitive should necessarily be treated by chemotherapy. A localized tumor that is equally radiosensitive or easily resectable can be cured by these methods without risking the *toxicity* of systemic therapy. On the other hand, chemotherapy may be the treatment of choice even though a tumor is relatively chemoinsensitive. Of course, there is no point in treating with a totally ineffective agent.

The similarities and differences in the effects of cell type on chemotherapy, as compared to radiotherapy, provide a starting point to a discussion of chemotherapeutic management. As previously described, response to radiotherapy can be predicted from the basic histologic cell type involved, i.e., lymphoma, carcinoma, sarcoma, and, in general, sensitivity decreases in that order. Within each of these groups some variation in sensitivity exists; however, available evidence indicates that site of origin has little effect on the radiosensitivity of the cell. For example, adenocarcinoma of the breast is of the same order of sensitivity as adenocarcinoma of the endometrium.

Sensitivity to chemotherapy has a similar overall pattern. In general, sensitivity of leukemias and lymphomas is greater than that of carcinomas and sarcomas. Within each of these groups some similarity in sensitivity exists, although adenocarcinomas usually exhibit greater sensitivity than squamous cell carcinomas. However, a significant difference in sensitivity to chemotherapy, as compared to radiotherapy, is found in the marked differences in sensitivity of histologically-alike tumors that have originated in different organs. For example, adenocarcinoma of the breast is one of the most chemosensitive tumors both in terms of cytotoxic drugs and hormonal manipulation, while adenocarcinoma of the endometrium is relatively hormonally responsive but poorly responsive to cytotoxic drugs and adenocarcinoma of the lung is poorly responsive to either. Thus, the ability to predict biologic response of a tumor *based on histology* may be accurate for radiotherapeutic, but not for chemotherapeutic management. Sensitivity to chemotherapy needs to be discussed in terms of a specific histologic cell type originating in a specific organ.

Cytotoxic Chemotherapy. In recent years, great progress has been achieved in the field of chemotherapy. Some tumors may now be controlled for many years, and it has become possible to speak of chemotherapeutic "cure." Unfortunately, at present, the list of diseases which respond so well is small, and none of the most common tumors, i.e., lung, breast, prostate, or colon, are on this list.

In the interest of clarity, only those tumors which show substantial benefit when treated by chemotherapy are discussed. The specific drug regimens described should be considered merely as examples of current therapy; other regimens are possible. In addition, results reflect aggressive care in expert hands and may not be reproducible universally.

As in other specialized disciplines, medical oncology has its own jargon, in particular, its own precise definitions of response. The effectiveness of chemotherapy is frequently measured by its ability to prolong survival, ameliorate symptoms or decrease tumor size. Unfortunately, it is never possible to demonstrate increased survival for any particular patient and the evaluation of improvement in symptoms is so subjective and poorly reproducible that measurement of objective criteria, such as tumor size, is the primary means by which drugs are evaluated. To facilitate intercomparison of results, definitions similar to the following are used. *Complete response*—complete disappearance of all measurable disease maintained for a given period of time. *Partial response*—decrease of at least 50% in the sum of the products of the greatest perpendicular diameters of all measurable disease, with no evidence of progression. *Response*—any decrease in size of the sum of the products of the greatest perpendicular diameters without evidence of progression.

DISEASES RESPONSIVE TO CHEMOTHERAPY

Choriocarcinoma. Choriocarcinoma in females is an unusual tumor that is related to trophoblastic growth. This is one of the few diseases that can be controlled even after metastases occur. At present, approximately 75% of high risk patients who present with metastases can be brought into prolonged, complete remission and 95 to 100% of patients who are treated in the early stages of disease experience complete remission.[15] In fact, chemotherapy is so efficient that adjunctive surgery usually is not necessary. Treatment of low risk patients requires treatment with one drug only (usually methotrexate) but high risk patients probably should receive combination chemotherapy.

Acute Lymphocytic Leukemia. Leukemia is the most common malignancy in children and acute lymphocytic leukemia is the most frequent type. Treatment of this disease is complex and requires multidrug regimens which are quite toxic and requires facilities where supportive care can be provided. Treatment is performed in several stages. Initially a remission must be induced. This is usually done with at least two drugs, vincristine and prednisone, and leads to complete remission in 80 to 90% of affected children. Because relapse can rapidly follow cessation of induction therapy, many physicians now try to consolidate this gain by subsequently adding other active agents such as L-asparaginase or daunomycin. Next, the central nervous system is treated separately because the previously mentioned agents do not effectively eradicate disease in this site. Low dose irradiation and intrathecal chemotherapy have each been used effectively for this purpose. Last, the patient is kept on maintenance therapy, usually with combinations such as methotrexate, 6-mercaptopurine, cytosine arabinoside and cyclophosphamide, for a period of time, although to date the optimum duration of maintenance therapy is unknown. With therapy as described above, 50% of treated children are surviving at least 5 years, free of disease.[16]

Hodgkin's Disease. Although radiotherapy is the treatment of choice for localized Hodgkin's disease, chemotherapy is indicated for advanced cases. Aggressive four-drug regimens are required (usually Mustard, Oncovin, Prednisone and Procarbazine) but long-term complete remissions are possible. In the original NCI study, 43 patients were given "MOPP" and 35 experienced complete remission of disease which persisted in 15 at a maximum follow-up of 52 months.[17] Subsequent studies have also demonstrated complete remissions in more than one half of patients with a substantial fraction remaining free of disease for extended periods.[18]

Testicular Carcinoma. While there is considerable debate concerning optimal treatment for the various stages of testicular carcinoma (teratocarcinoma, embryonal cell carcinoma and choriocarcinoma), there is little doubt that multidrug regimens can produce substantial response rates.[19] For example, Einhorn et al.[20] reported the preliminary results of treatment by a three-drug regimen (bleomycin, vinblastine and cis-platinum). Of 20 evaluable patients, 15 experienced complete regression with 13 remaining disease-free from 6 to 18 months.

Non-Hodgkin's Lymphoma. The non-Hodgkin's lymphomas are more than a group of tumors that are not quite Hodgkin's disease. In terms of behavior, prognosis and response to treatment (including chemotherapy), they are unique. In fact, each of the non-Hodgkin's lymphomas has slightly different behavior and prognosis than the others.

Several classification systems for non-Hodgkin's lymphomas are in use. The most common, the Rappaport system, divides them into nine histologic types which also correlate with behavior and prognosis. Tumors are classified by their overall architecture (nodular or diffuse patterns) and by their predominant cell type (lymphocytic well-differentiated, lymphocytic poorly-differentiated, mixed, "histiocytic," and undifferentiated) (Fig. 5–3).

Within this system, nodular tumors are less aggressive than diffuse tumors and lymphocytic tumors are less aggressive than histiocytic

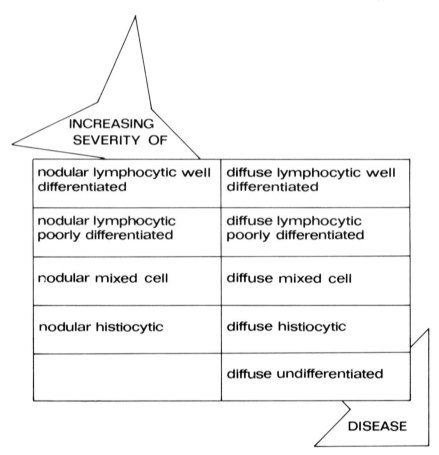

Fig. 5–3. *Types of non-Hodgkin's lymphoma. Disease types in upper left corner are less aggressive than those in lower right corner.*

tumors. Consequently, those tumors depicted in the upper left hand corner of Figure 5–3 recur at a slower rate and have a better prognosis than those tumors in the lower right hand corner of the figure. In addition, when a patient with nodular lymphocytic disease relapses, the disease can more frequently be brought back into remission than can diffuse histiocytic disease. On the other hand, relatively short-term complete response rates more accurately reflect the value of chemotherapy (or radiotherapy) for diffuse histiocytic lymphomas than for nodular lymphocytic disease, because few recurrences occur after 2 years in diffuse histiocytic, while delayed recurrence is the rule with nodular lymphocytic poorly differentiated disease.

The manner in which chemotherapy is given for the non-Hodgkin's lymphomas reflects both this biologic behavior and chemosensitivity. Nodular disease can be treated "gently" with a single agent (usually cyclophosphamide) and treatment yields 30 to 50% complete response rates.[21] Nonetheless, the most common regimen has been a three-drug combination of cyclophosphamide, vincristine and prednisone. Such combinations produce complete responses in approximately 40% of advanced non-Hodgkin's lymphomas.[22] Some groups are now adding bleomycin and/or adriamycin to this regimen for histiocytic disease and are reporting patients with disease-free survival beyond a 2-year period, after which few recurrences are expected.

Multiple Myeloma. Multiple myeloma is a hematologic neoplasm characterized by excessive proliferation of plasma cells. These cells retain their ability to produce immunoglobulin, and the hallmark of the disease is therefore hyperglobulinemia. The excessive proliferation affects bone marrow, kidneys, cortical bone and blood, causing a myriad of signs and symptoms. Early in the course of disease, only hyperglobulinemia may be present, and no therapy is indicated until progression is evident. When required, chemotherapy usually consists of two agents, melphalan and prednisone.[23] With this regimen, approximately 50 to 70% of patients experience objective response (including decrease in globulins and calcium and increase in hemoglobin), although recalcification of lytic bone lesions is rare and adjuvant palliative radiotherapy to such lesions is not infrequently required. Prolongation of survival has also been reported.

Breast. In females, adenocarcinomas of the breast account for the most frequent cause of cancer-related deaths. However, many breast cancers behave in a far less aggressive fashion, and in clinical practice, one must be able to distinguish between the various forms of the disease; a prememopausal woman in whom disease recurs in multiple anatomic sites within a few months of diagnosis has a very different disease than an elderly woman in whom disease recurs only on the chest wall, many years after primary treatment. In the former case, death usually occurs in a matter of months, while in the latter, many years of useful life in symbiosis with disease typically occur.

As might be expected, therapy should be matched to the individual behavior of disease. In general, cytotoxic chemotherapy is required for aggressive presentations while hormonal management (Chap. 6) and/or local radiotherapy will suffice for non-threatening disease. Even within the category of cytotoxic therapy, there is a wide range of effective drugs and regimens, and the inherent risk of any regimen must be weighed against the risk of not controlling the tumor rapidly.

Single agent chemotherapy is possible with a wide variety of agents but recently has fallen into general disfavor. More commonly used are combination regimens, with the prototype of such treatment being the three-drug combination of cyclophosphamide, methotrexate and 5-fluorouracil. Such regimens provide substantial regression of disease in approximately one-half of patients, including complete regression in about 15%.[24]

Ovary. Ovarian carcinoma infrequently is diagnosed early and at times cannot be resected. In addition, recurrent disease occurs in at least one-third of seemingly totally resected cases. Unlike many tumors, ovarian cancer tends to recur locally, within the abdomen, rather than as distant metastases.

Chemotherapy classically has employed single agents such as melphalan. Such treatment yields response in about one-half of cases which persists for 2 years in approximately 10% of patients.[25] Recently multidrug regimens have been studied, and at least one prospective trial indicates improvement in response rates with such therapy.[26]

Adjuvant Therapy. Just as combinations of drugs have yielded improved results, combinations of surgery, radiotherapy and chemotherapy have significantly improved results in some diseases. In general, the greatest advances have come about by the use of adjuvant treatment, before the tumor has had the opportunity to recur. Carcinoma of the breast has received most of the publicity, but this approach was pioneered for pediatric tumors and has provided significant gains against these diseases. Because therapy is administered without proof of disease, response rates cannot be measured and such treatment is therefore described elsewhere (Chap. 10).

References

1. Maier, J.G., Sulak, M.H., and Mittemeyer, B.T.: Seminomas of the Testes: Analysis of Treatment Success and Failure. A.J.R. *102*:596–602, 1968.
2. Doornbos, J.F., Hussey, D.H., and Johnson, D.E.: Radiotherapy for Pure Seminoma of the Testes. Radiology *116*:401–404, 1975.
3. Kaplan, H.S.: Evidence for a Tumoricidal Dose Level in the Radiotherapy of Hodgkin's Disease. Cancer Res. *26*: 1221–1224, 1966.
4. ———: *Hodgkin's Disease*, Cambridge, Harvard University Press, 1972.
5. Bush, R.S., et al.: Radiation Therapy of Localized Non-Hodgkin's Lymphoma. Cancer Treat. Rep. *61*:1129–1136, 1977.

6. Helman, S., et al.: The Place of Radiation Therapy in the Treatment of Non-Hodgkin's Lymphomas. Cancer 39:843–851, 1977.
7. Caldwell, W.L.: Carcinoma of the Urinary Bladder. J.A.M.A. 229:1643–1645, 1974.
8. Goffinet, D.R., et al.: Bladder Cancer: Results of Radiation Therapy in 384 Patients. Radiology 117:149–153, 1975.
9. Pearson, J.G.: The Present Status and Future Potential of Radiotherapy in the Management of Esophageal Cancer. Cancer 39:882–890, 1977.
10. Suit, H.D., and Russell, W.O.: Soft Part Tumors. Cancer 39:830–836, 1977.
11. Edland, R.W.: Liposarcoma—A Retrospective Study of 15 Cases, A Review of the Literature and a Discussion of Radiosensitivity. A.J.R. 103:778–791, 1967.
12. Windeyer, B., Dische, S., and Mansfield, C.M.: The Place of Radiotherapy in the Management of Fibrosarcoma of the Soft Tissues. Clin. Rad. 17:32–40, 1966.
13. Cassady, J.R., et al.: Radiation Therapy for Rhabdomyosarcoma. Radiology 91:116–120, 1968.
14. Hornsey, S.: The Relationship Between Total Dose, Number of Fractions and Fraction Size in the Response of Malignant Melanoma in Patients. Br. J. Radiol. 51:905–909, 1978.
15. Lewis, J.L.: Current Status of Treatment of Gestational Trophoblastic Disease. Cancer 38:620–626, 1976.
16. Simone, J.V., et al.: Modality Therapy of Acute Lymphocytic Leukemia. Cancer 35:25–35, 1975.
17. Devita, V.E.T., Serpick, A.A., and Carbone, P.P.: Combination Chemotherapy in the Treatment of Advanced Hodgkin's Disease. Ann. Intern. Med. 73:881–895, 1970.
18. Goldsmith, M.A., and Carter, S.K.: Combination Chemotherapy of Advanced Hodgkin's Disease. Cancer 33:1–8, 1974.
19. Carter, S.K., and Wasserman, T.H.: The Chemotherapy of Urologic Cancer. Cancer 36:729–747, 1975.
20. Einhorn, L.H., Furnass, B.E., and Powell, N.: Combination Chemotherapy of Disseminated Testicular Carcinoma with Cis-platinum Diammine Dichloride (CPDD), Vinblastine (VLB), and Bleomycin (BLEO). Proceedings of the Amer. Soc. Clin. Oncol., 17:240, 1976.
21. Jones, S.E., et al.: Non-Hodgkin's Lymphomas—II. Single Agent Chemotherapy. Cancer 30:31–38, 1972.
22. Schein, P.S., et al.: Results of Combination Chemotherapy of Non-Hodgkin's Lymphoma. Br. J. Cancer 31:465–473, 1975.
23. Alexanian, R., et al.: Treatment for Multiple Myeloma. J.A.M.A. 208:1680–1685, 1969.
24. Canellos, G.P., et al.: Combination Chemotherapy for Metastatic Breast Carcinoma. Cancer 38:1882–1886, 1976.
25. Young, R.C.: Chemotherapy of Ovarian Cancer: Past and Present. Semin. Oncol. 2:267–276, 1975.
26. Young, R.C., et al.: Advanced Ovarian Adenocarcinoma. N. Engl. J. Med. 299:1261–1266, 1978.

6

EFFECT OF
DIFFERENTIATION

Differentiation has several meanings. In reference to normal cells it implies specialization of function; the ability to perform specific tasks not done by most other cells. Neural cells "think," pneumocytes exchange gases, pancreatic cells produce enzymes, and so forth. Each of these cells differentiates from the same original cell and, presumably, contains identical genetic material, but each expresses only a part of its genetic constitution.

Differentiation also applies to histologic appearance. Cells not only have various functions, they have various shapes and growth patterns. Neural tissue, lung tissue and pancreatic tissue, for example, are quite dissimilar in appearance. On the other hand, cells which perform similar functions tend to have similar appearances. Thus histologic differentiation and functional differentiation are not unrelated.

Equally important is what the differentiated cell is *not*. Implicit in specialization is the loss of other cellular functions. The differentiated cell cannot function autonomously. It must rely on other cells to supply some of its needs and the needs of the organism as a whole. Most notably, the specialized cell normally does not proliferate. Differentiation in normal tissues then, describes the change from an immature pleuripotent, proliferative cell to a mature, specialized, non-proliferative cell. The term differentiation is applied quite differently to tumors.

Cellular Differentiation of Tumors. In reference to tumors, differentiation describes the degree to which the tumor retains the functional or histologic characteristics of its parent normal tissue. Functionally this can be manifest as sensitivity to hormonal stimuli, as may

103

occur in carcinoma of the breast, or as the ability to perform a specialized function, as may occur with a thyroid carcinoma which concentrates iodine. When function is involved, description is relatively simple. The cell either can or cannot perform a task normally done by its parent tissue. If it can, some indication of the degree to which function has been retained is indicated, but in most instances a qualitative description will suffice. For example, a particular tumor may be described as being highly, moderately, or only slightly responsive to hormonal control.

Description of differentiation on morphologic grounds is more complex. While the same general rules apply (i.e., those cells which retain the features of their parent tissue are considered well-differentiated), the specific histologic criteria used for this determination vary according to the type of tumor. Several classification systems exist, such as the Broders system for epithelial lesions and the Kernohan system for brain tumors. Sometimes numerical grades (I-III or I-IV) are given, while at other times qualitative descriptions suffice, but in any case, low grade well-differentiated tumors resemble their parent tissue while high grade, poorly-differentiated tumors do not. Although complete discussion of the criteria a pathologist uses to designate the degree of differentiation are beyond the scope of this book, some basic guidelines are presented.

Epithelial Tumors. The epithelial tumors, squamous cell and adenocarcinomas are derived from cells which cover internal and external surfaces of the body. Squamous cells have flattened shape and produce keratin, while adenomatous cells are arranged in gland-like formations. The degree to which a tumor exhibits these characteristics determines its differentiation.

Squamous tumors are termed well-differentiated when the cells are of uniform appearance, show few mitotic figures, produce keratin and are arranged in circular nests called "epithelial pearls." At the other end of the spectrum, poorly-differentiated squamous tumors have a non-uniform pattern of cells with many in mitosis (some abnormal), and produce no keratin.

Well-differentiated adenocarcinomas exhibit an orderly pattern of cells in glandular formations. There are few mitotic figures and histologic differences from normal glands are subtle. Poorly-differentiated lesions, on the other hand, are disorderly with little tendency toward gland formation and have many mitotic figures, some abnormal. At times, the tumor is barely recognizable as an adenocarcinoma and at other times, electron microscopy is required to establish a histologic diagnosis.

Sarcomas. Sarcomas arise from tissues of mesodermal origin such as muscle, fat and connective tissue, and display a wide variety of histologic appearances. While the basic concept of grading applies to these lesions, the variety of histologic appearances precludes simple rules for description. In addition, differentiation generally is of less prognostic value for sarcoma than carcinoma. For example, some aggressive chondrosarcomas have cartilage cells which appear nearly normal, while some benign diseases have an appearance similar to aggressive sarcomas.

Even so, subdivision is possible and of some value. Liposarcomas, for instance, come in well-differentiated, myxoid, round cell and pleomorphic variants. Other sarcomas have similar categories. Prognostically, at least for some sarcomas, the number of mitoses is a useful feature. Ten mitoses per 10 high power microscopic fields appears to be a useful yardstick; lesions that exhibit fewer than 10 tend to be less aggressive than those with more.

Brain Tumors. The majority of brain tumors are composed of neoplastic glial cells. These tumors range from the well-differentiated astrocytoma characterized by a slight increase in cellularity to the anaplastic glioblastoma with its cellular pleomorphism, frequent mitoses, necrosis and hemorrhage.

The Lymphomas. As previously described, lymphomas are divided into two major categories, Hodgkin's and non-Hodgkin's lymphoma. Within both categories, there are several subtypes which, in effect, are somewhat analogous to various degrees of differentiation. However, it should be noted that they represent *varying architectural patterns of the tumor,* as well as *different stages in the maturational process of lymphocytes,* rather than degrees of resemblance to a parent tissue. Within the category of Hodgkin's lymphomas, lymphocyte predominant disease is the equivalent of well-differentiated tumor, while lymphocyte depleted disease is akin to a poorly-differentiated lesion. As noted in Chapter 5, *nodular lymphocytic well-differentiated* disease and *diffuse undifferentiated* disease form opposite ends of the spectrum of non-Hodgkin's lymphoma.

Differentiation vs. Site of Disease. The degree of differentiation of a tumor is not unpredictable. Despite the legion of known carcinogens and the probable large number of as yet unknown carcinogens, the spectrum of differentiation at any site is remarkably constant. Thus, the site of disease, not the cause, appears to be a primary determinant of differentiation. This implies that cancer induction is not a totally random change as random change should lead to similar spectra of differentiation at all anatomic sites. Such is definitely not the case. While tumors of any degree of differentiation can occur at any site, the following associations hold true overall.

Well-differentiated Tumors. Well-differentiated tumors occur frequently among many kinds of neoplasms including carcinomas of the skin, lip, oral cavity, endometrium, prostate, penis and vulva (labia). Certain sites also appear to be predisposed to formation of the well-differentiated form of tumors which occur in other degrees of differentiation elsewhere. For example, cerebellar tumors in children tend to be well-differentiated astrocytomas and mediastinal Hodgkin's disease tends to be of the nodular sclerosing type.

Poorly-differentiated Tumors. Neoplasms arising in the nasopharynx, hypopharynx and esophagus tend to be poorly differentiated. Again, a selective influence of the site of disease exists. For example, non-Hodgkin's lymphoma arising in bone is almost always histocytic.

Implications of Differentiation. No specific morphologic feature, including the degree of differentiation, should be used by itself to predict the biologic behavior or efficacy of therapy of tumors. Such predictions must be based on the entire clinical picture including type, extent, differentiation and previous treatment of the tumor as well as age, sex, general health status, and habits of the host. Nevertheless, each of these factors influences management to a degree, and if taken in the proper perspective—as a guide and not as an absolute—can be helpful.

Effect of Differentiation on Sensitivity to Treatment. The effect of cellular differentiation on the likely response to radiotherapy has been discussed for many years. In 1906, Bergonié and Tribondeau codified their beliefs in the form of a "law" which bears their name. Translated from the original French, the law states that "the effect of radiations on living cells is the more intense: (1) the greater their reproductive activity, (2) the longer their mitotic phase lasts and (3) the less their morphology and function are differentiated."[1] The first two factors are based on changes in radiosensitivity which occur during the cell cycle and will be discussed in Chapter 8. The validity of the last factor is examined here.

Rate of Response. Intensity of effect generally has been translated as rate of regression. In general, the more *un*differentiated the lesion, the more rapidly it will respond to treatment. However, some well-differentiated tumors, such as seminomas, are obvious exceptions to this rule.

Radiosensitivity vs. Rate of Response. As described in Chapter 5, cellular radiosensitivity is measured by the slope of the survival curve. Rate of regression of tumor plays no part in this description. On the other hand, through the years, both radiotherapists and non-radiotherapists have been impressed by, and sought to describe, variations in rate of regression of different tumors. Because tumors that disappeared quickly usually were controlled, at least locally, this association led to the improper description of such tumors as sensitive. Conversely, tumors which did not regress rapidly were thought insensitive. The descriptions have persisted in some circles. It is not unusual for a referring physician to question the need for completion of the entire planned course of therapy when a tumor disappears quickly. Alternatively, aggressive surgery is occasionally suggested when a lesion fails to resolve rapidly during treatment.

Several authors have recently presented data indicating that rate of response does not predict eventual outcome. Suit et al.[2] reviewed the clinical course of patients who received therapeutic irradiation for advanced squamous cell carcinoma of the oropharynx. Correlation between rate of tumor regression and local tumor control was not evident. Sobel et al.[3] measured tumor clearance or persistence at varying times, during and after radiotherapy, for a large group of patients who had squamous cell carcinoma of the oral cavity, oropharynx or hypopharynx. Rate of regression was less important in determining eventual control than was the presence or absence of disease 2 to 3 months after completion of therapy. However, even when clinical examination at 2 to 3 months revealed residual induration (which was interpreted as evidence of persistent disease) 25 to 35% of patients eventually proved to be locally free of disease.

Marcial and Bosch[4] examined the rate of regression of irradiated cervical carcinomas. In advanced disease, continued shrinkage occurred for several months after completion of treatment and in some cases, up to 10 months passed before disease completely resolved. No correlation between the interval required for regression and the incidence of permanent local control was evident. Interestingly, histologic grade did not influence the rate of response.

At other sites regression may be even slower. Rider[5] has reported 65 patients treated by radiotherapy alone for inoperable carcinoma of the rectum below the peritoneal reflection. Survival at 5 years was 29%, twice the rate found in a matched group with less advanced operable disease treated by abdomenoperineal resection. However, many of these patients required a year or more for disease to regress completely as measured by digital rectal examination or needle biopsy. In fact, Rider advises against intervention as long as the disease is either stable or regressing after therapy, no matter how slowly.

In summary, although the degree of differentiation *may* predict rate of response, rate of response neither determines radiosensitivity nor outcome of treatment. Despite this, degree of differentiation does affect therapy and prognosis.

Relation of Differentiation to Biologic Behavior. As discussed previously, cell type is the primary determinant of tumor behavior; however, the degree of cellular differentiation is an important modifying influence. In general, the more poorly differentiated the tumor, the more aggressive its behavior. Local, regional and distant spread increases, recurrence rate increases, and survival decreases as grade increases. DeSaia et al.[6] present data, collected from the literature, illustrating this concept. For endometrial carcinoma, as differentiation deteriorates through grades 1, 2 and 3, deep myometrial invasion increases from 8 to 20 to 44% and survival decreases from 82 to 75 to 43%. Similar data are available for other types of tumor. This relation must be respected when considering treatment.

At times degree of differentiation may be the deciding factor. For example, transurethral resection for benign prostatic hypertrophy occasionally reveals occult adenocarcinoma. In general, such lesions are well-differentiated, do not progress rapidly, and even if untreated, do not decrease life expectancy.[7,8] However, if these lesions are undifferentiated, they behave in an aggressive manner and are rarely cured even by radical prostatectomy in expert hands.[9] Thus, the degree of differentiation, by predicting biologic behavior, at times dictates the need (or lack of need) for active therapy.

Exploiting Differentiation. In addition to their relatively non-aggressive behavior, well-differentiated tumors sometimes provide the physician with unique opportunities for diagnosis and/or treatment. Two manifestations of differentiation have been exploited clinically: (1) the ability to selectively concentrate iodine, as may occur in thyroid carcinoma, and (2) the ability to respond to hormonal stimuli, as may occur in breast, endometrial and prostatic carcinomas.

[131]I and Thyroid Carcinoma. Normal thyroid tissue readily concentrates and stores iodine. Some thyroid tumors partially retain this ability, although they almost never function as well as their parent tissue. Follicular thyroid tumors most closely resemble normal tissue and most often concentrate substantial amounts of iodine; anaplastic thyroid tumors rarely concentrate even minimal amounts. Because the mechanism by which iodine is trapped and stored cannot distinguish between various isotopes of iodine (all isotopes of any element behave identically in chemical reactions), if a radioactive isotope, such as ^{131}I comes into contact with functioning thyroid tissue (normal or malignant) it will be retained. These principles form the theoretical basis for ^{131}I thyroid scanning, whole body scanning and isotope therapy.

Thyroid scans are radiographic images of the functional capacity of the gland. In practice, a minute quantity of ^{131}I is ingested by the patient, and, after a suitable interval, each part of the thyroid is scanned for retained radioactivity. Areas of normal tissue acquire approximately equal amounts of radioactivity but areas of abnormal tissue, either benign or malignant, may acquire greater or lesser amounts. The scan detects these variations in levels of radioactivity and records them on film. By convention relatively high levels of activity appear dark, or "hot" while low levels appear light, or "cold." However, cold regions on scans do not necessarily represent tumor. In fact, depending on the age, sex and diet of the patients who are being scanned, only about 20% of cold nodules are malignant. Uncommonly, a distinct hot area appears on a scan; such lesions nearly always are benign. While this examination is based on the relative inability of thyroid tumors to concentrate iodine, diagnosis and therapy of metastatic thyroid carcinomas benefit from the ability of some thyroid tumors to concentrate even limited amounts of iodine.

Although carcinoma of the thyroid (except for the anaplastic variants) usually behaves in a slowly progressive fashion, metastases to bone and lung do occur. Most patients with metastatic disease previously have been treated for their primary tumor—sometimes by total thyroidectomy. In such patients the tumor does not have to compete with normal thyroid tissue for iodine, and, if radioiodine is administered, sufficient amounts may concentrate in metastases to be detectable. A whole body scan demonstrates the location of these metastases as relatively hot areas against a non-radioactive background. If the patient has metastases and still has functioning normal thyroid, ablation either by surgery (preferably) or irradiation is necessary before substantial uptake of iodine by metastases can be expected. In this manner, Henk et al.[10] were able to detect distant metastases from thyroid carcinoma in 4 of 9 patients who, despite other radiographic procedures, were thought to have disease confined to the neck.

In some patients, well-differentiated metastases take up radioiodine so avidly that the trapped radioactivity destroys (or at least damages) the metastases while causing only minimal damage to the surrounding normal tissue. This forms the basis for ^{131}I therapy.

From Pochin's experience[11,12] it appears that about 80% of patients who have well-differentiated thyroid tumors which have inoperable spread are suitable candidates for radioiodine therapy and of these, 50% will have an excellent response and an additional 25% should experience some palliation. Harness et al.[13] found that such therapy substantially improves survival. Of 36 patients who had metastatic pulmonary and/or osseous spread from well-differentiated thyroid carcinomas, only 28% of patients died of their metastases after radioiodine therapy (average follow-up 15 years), which the authors compared to a 75% mortality of similar patients (at 5 years) reported by others.

Hormonal Therapy. Hormones are chemicals influencing behavior of body organs. In normal circumstances, they provide a mechanism for adjustment and control. Tumors derived from organs which respond to or depend on hormonal control, may retain this dependence. In such cases, hormonal manipulation can be used to influence the course of disease.

Although many organs are normally responsive to hormonal stimuli, three types of tumors, endometrial, prostatic and breast, account for the vast majority of cases where hormonal control is of clinical benefit. Addition, subtraction and inhibition of hormones can all be used, and recently, assays to predict the likelihood of response to such manipulation, have become part of clinical practice.

Some general comments about hormonal therapy are in order. Regression of disease results from physiologic changes not cytotoxicity, and it is, therefore, illogical to hope for total tumor destruction. If the intention of therapy is cure of disease, hormonal therapy by itself is inappropriate. On the other hand, hormonal therapy is usually less toxic to normal cells, and when applicable, has a distinct advantage over cytotoxic chemotherapy by inducing regression of disease without inducing myelosuppression, and so forth. This is not to say that hormonal therapy is totally without side effects. For example, estrogen therapy not infrequently will produce nausea and vomiting, and more important, occasionally induces hypercalcemia. Fortunately, such changes are rapidly reversible with cessation of therapy.

In addition, because hormonal therapy relies on physiologic change, the process is slow and a minimum of 6 to 8 weeks of therapy usually is required to obtain results. Thus, it should not be used in life-threatening situations.

Hormonal Therapy of Endometrial Carcinoma. The cyclic variation in growth of uterine endometrium during the normal menstrual cycle is well known. Early in the cycle, the influence of estrogen is high and the endometrium hypertrophies; late in the cycle, progesterone levels peak and the endometrium involutes. It required only a small step in logic to apply this concept to neoplastic disease to try to induce regression of metastases from endometrial carcinoma by progestational agents.

Kelley and Baker[14] reviewed the literature concerning progesterone therapy of metastatic endometrial carcinoma. Response rates of approximately 30% were noted, with the most frequent responses being seen in well-differentiated tumors. Such therapy is particularly efficacious for slowly growing pulmonary metastases.

Hormonal Therapy of Prostatic Carcinoma. Although it hardly seems sufficient compensation, it is a fact that eunuchs are not afflicted by prostatic carcinoma. Thus, the growth of prostatic carcinoma appears to depend on circulating androgens and the treatment of symptomatic prostatic metastases by orchiectomy is both logical and effective. Less easily explained is the approximately equal chance of control by administration of estrogens. The Veterans Administration Cooperative Urologic Research Group[15] randomized patients with distant metastases from prostate carcinoma and treated by (1) orchiectomy, (2) estrogens, (3) orchiectomy plus estrogens or (4) placebo. This study revealed a slight advantage for the orchiectomy group although much, if not all, of this advantage over the estrogen group was secondary to the induction of cardiovascular deaths by the dose of estrogen used. The smaller dose of estrogen in current use appears to be equally effective against tumor and less likely to produce cardiovascular problems. No advantage for combined use of orchiectomy and estrogen was evident, and it is mentioned only to be condemned. Selection between orchiectomy and estrogen therapy can be made depending on the individual preference of the patient. For those cases going to be treated by estrogen, low dose irradiation of the breasts prevents subsequent gynecomastia.

Hormone Treatment of Breast Cancer. For several reasons treatment of metastatic breast cancer with hormones is complex. *First*, breast cancer can respond to a variety of hormonal agents and treatments: estrogens, androgens, anti-estrogens, oophorectomy, adrenalectomy and hypophysectomy. *Second*, response is modified by the menstrual status of the patient. *Third*, breast cancer behaves in a wide variety of ways; hormonal therapy is appropriate for only some of them. *Fourth*, the likely efficacy of hormone therapy must be weighed against alternative treatment modalities: analgesics, radiotherapy, surgery or cytotoxic chemotherapy. Fortunately, it is now possible to pre-select those patients who are likely to benefit from hormonal therapy based on hormone receptor protein analyses.

Estrogens can be considered the "standard" hormone therapy. Response is most frequent in postmenopausal women, perhaps because their tumors grow in a relatively estrogen-deficient environment, and averages approximately 35%.[16] In premenopausal women the rate is considerably lower and such therapy risks exacerbating disease. Estrogens are most effective against soft tissue metastases and relatively ineffective against visceral disease. In addition, some patients who transiently respond to estrogen therapy have a secondary response to subsequent estrogen withdrawal.

The counterpart of adding estrogens for postmenopausal disease is removing them for premenopausal disease. Castration leads to regression of disease in 40% of such patients[16] and is preferably accomplished by surgical oophorectomy. For patients who refuse surgery, low dose irradiation of the ovaries will yield equivalent results but requires more time for response to occur. Patients who receive substantial transient benefit from oophorectomy, upon relapse, can be considered for secondary ablative procedures such as adrenalectomy or hypophysectomy to further decrease circulating estrogen levels.

The administration of androgens might seem to provide a simple antagonist to estrogenic action. There is little doubt that such therapy sometimes is effective. Even so, Kennedy[17] has found evidence in the literature that 21% of postmenopausal women respond to androgens, at a time when they should have little circulatory estrogen to oppose. In addition, it can be shown that androgens are metabolically converted into estrogens to some degree. Recently, true anti-estrogen compounds have become available. With these drugs response rates approximating 30% have been reported.[18] Interestingly, the drugs are effective in both pre- and postmenopausal patients and appear to work only in those patients who would respond to "classical" methods.

Thus, the selection of appropriate hormonal management requires some clinical experience. Fortunately, an assay of the ability of breast cancer cells to manufacture an estrogen receptor protein is now available. The presence of this protein suggests that the tumor, like normal breast cells, responds to hormonal manipulation and appears to be equally accurate in predicting whether estrogen is added or subtracted. McGuire[19] reviewed the literature and found 55 to 60% response rate to manipulation in estrogen receptor positive (ER+) patients but only about a 5% response when this protein was absent. Unfortunately, the presence or absence of protein is not an all-or-none phenomenon, and the predictive ability of this test appears to depend on the *quantitative* level of protein used to call the assay positive. In addition, other receptor proteins influence response. Degenshein et al.[20] have studied progesterone receptor proteins and reported 6 responses in 7 ER+, PR+ patients, 0 in 5 ER+, PR− patients, and 0 in 4 ER−, PR− patients treated by ablative surgery.

References

1. Del Regato, J.A., and Spjut, H.J.: *Cancer—Diagnosis, Treatment, and Prognosis*. 5th Ed., St. Louis, The C.V. Mosby Co., 1977, p. 73.
2. Suit, H.D., Lindberg, R.D., and Fletcher, G.H.: Prognostic Significance of Extent of Tumor Regression at Completion of Radiation Therapy. Radiology *84*:1100–1107, 1965.
3. Sobel, S., *et al.*: Tumor Persistence As A Predictor of Outcome After Radiation Therapy of Head and Neck Cancers. Int. J. Rad. Oncol., Biol., Phys. *1*:873–880, 1976.
4. Marcial, V.A., and Bosch, A.: Radiation-Induced Tumor Regression in Carcinoma of the Uterine Cervix: Prognostic Significance. Am. J. Roent. *108*:113–123, 1970.
5. Rider, W.D.: Is the Miles Operation Really Necessary for the Treatment of Rectal Cancer? J. Can. Assoc. Rad. *26*:167–175, 1975.
6. DiSaia, P.J., Morrow, C.P., and Townsend, D.E.: *Synopsis of Gynecologic Oncology*. New York, John Wiley and Sons, 1975, pp. 111–135.
7. Whitmore, W.F.: The Natural History of Prostatic Cancer. Cancer *32*:1104–1112, 1973.

8. Byar, D.P., and the V. A. Cooperative Urological Research Group: Survival of Patients with Incidentally Found Microscopic Cancer of the Prostate: Results of a Clinical Trial of Conservative Treatment. J. Urol. *108*:908–913, 1972.

9. Del Regato, J.A., and Spjut, H.J.: *Cancer—Diagnosis, Treatment and Prognosis.* 5th Ed., St. Louis, The C. V. Mosby Co., 1977, p. 668.

10. Henk, J.M., Kirkman, S., and Owen, G.M.: Whole-body Scanning and [131]I Therapy in the Management of Thyroid Carcinoma. Br. J. Radiol. *45*:369–376, 1972.

11. Pochin, E.E.: Radioiodine Therapy of Thyroid Cancer. Semin. Nucl. Med. *1*:503–515, 1971.

12. Pochin, E.E.: Prospects from the Treatment of Thyroid Carcinoma with Radioiodine. Clin. Rad. *18*:113–135, 1967.

13. Harness, J.K., et al.: Differentiated Thyroid Carcinomas—Treatment of Distant Metastases. Arch. Surg. *108*:410–419, 1974.

14. Kelley, R.M., and Baker, W.H.: The Role of Progesterone in Human Endometrial Cancer. Cancer Res. *25*:1190–1192, 1965.

15. The V. A. Cooperative Urological Research Group: Treatment and Survival of Patients with Cancer of the Prostate. Surg. Gyn. Obstet. *124*:1011–1017, 1967.

16. Kennedy, B.J.: Hormonal Therapies in Breast Cancer. Sem. Oncol. *1*:119–130, 1974.

17. ———: Hormonal Therapy for Advanced Breast Cancer. Cancer *18*:1551–1557, 1965.

18. Legha, S.S., Slavik, M., and Carter, S.K.: Nafoxidine—An Antiestrogen for the Treatment of Breast Cancer. Cancer *38*:1535–1541, 1976.

19. McGuire, W.L.: Current Status of Estrogen Receptors in Human Breast Cancer. Cancer *36*:638–644, 1975.

20. Degenshein, G.A., et al.: Estrogen and Progesterone Receptor Site Studies as Guides to the Management of Advanced Breast Cancer. Breast; Diseases of the Breast *3*:29–31, 1977.

7

CELL CHANGES
SECONDARY TO
TREATMENT

Treatment by radiation and/or drugs has the intention of and capacity to injure cells. Several levels and possibly several types of injury occur, the degree and type being dependent upon cell type, radiation or drug type, rate at which treatment is given, dose of radiation or drug and physiologic state of the cell.

Sublethal and Lethal Injury. During and after any treatment by either radiation or cytotoxic drugs, some cells are killed, but there are a number of survivors too. Of the survivors, some may have been lucky and were uninjured because, for whatever reason, neither radiation nor drug harmed them. Others, however, may have been injured but the *level* of injury was too low to kill them. Thus, two general *levels* of cellular injury can be recognized; lethal and *sub*lethal. Among the sublethal injuries are several *types*, including mutations, malignant transformations and broken chromosomes. These sublethal injuries are the very ones which can lead to complications of radiation and/or drug exposure. Mutations have impact on the human population, malignant transformation can lead to cancer induction in treated persons, and chromosome abnormalities lead, among other things, to a number of birth defects. All of these changes will be discussed in greater detail later in this book.

Another type of damage affects cells' *reproductive apparatus*. If enough radiation or drug is given (under the right conditions), the reproductive apparatus is so badly damaged that cells lose the potential to reproduce. They become sterile and radiation or drug produced sterility is really the equivalent of a lethal injury. A sterile cell may live for a while but when the end of its life comes, it will die without having produced descendants.

Tumors are destroyed by irradiation or cytotoxic drugs because treatment using these modalities sterilizes parts of the tumor cell population. These sterile cells die in time and the tumor shrinks. The amount by which tumor shrinks, unfortunately, is rarely if ever equal to the volume occupied by the sterile cells. Uninjured or *sub*lethally injured cells multiply even as sterile cells are dying and to a greater or lesser degree, replace them. Shrinkage occurs when more cells· are made sterile than are produced by multiplication of "fertile" cells.

Promotion of Lethal Injury. Of course, the objective of cancer therapy is to kill—or to prevent from multiplying—cancer cells, without, at the same time killing too many normal cells. The most straightforward way of accomplishing this aim is to deliver a higher dose of whatever agent is used to the cancer than is delivered to normal tissues. With radiation therapy it is possible to realize this objective reasonably well. External beams (Cobalt-60 gamma rays, electron beams, x rays) can be shaped, and a relatively high, uniform dose can be given tumors, while substantially lesser doses are inflicted upon reasonably small amounts of neighboring normal tissues. Radiation also can be delivered to well-circumscribed volumes by surgically implanting interstitial radiation sources, which largely spare surrounding normal tissues.

On the other hand, chemotherapy *usually* is administered systemically so that delivering a higher dose to cancer than to normal tissue usually is not possible. Systemically administered drugs eventually reach most, if not all, cells and in not-too-different concentrations.

Exposure to Radiation. As has already been noted, radiation doses which fail to kill cells nonetheless have a probability of injuring them in a number of ways, but there appears to be a limit beyond which cells cannot tolerate sublethal damage. In fact, cell *killing* by radiation is believed by many authorities to be the result of accumulation of sufficient degrees of sublethal injury to prohibit life. In other words, commonly used radiations do not often kill mammalian cells by the production of a single event which is lethal. On the contrary, as radiations pass through cells they probably have to cause a number of injuries. When the *number* is high enough, injured cells die, but if the number is not high enough, injured cells live. Much depends on what has been injured. DNA (deoxyribonucleic acid) damaged by radiation is believed to be *potentially* lethal; DNA is reparable, but evidently the repair process takes some time. If cells can repair damaged DNA *before* they must divide, chances are they will survive. However, if damaged DNA is not repaired before division, the injury is likely to be lethal. Clearly, post-irradiation activity of DNA-damaged cells is quite important. It can make the difference between cellular survival or death. In mitotically static tissues it seems reasonable to surmise that fewer cells will be killed by given radiation doses than in mitotically active ones, because potentially lethal DNA lesions will be permitted sufficient time to be repaired in many cells. It is well to note, however, that repair of DNA may not always be perfect; errors are occasionally made and these errors can lead to mutations. Given doses of radiation may kill more cells in mitotically active tissues than in static ones (because of the larger number that fail to repair potentially lethal DNA injuries), but larger numbers of mutations may be harbored in static tissues than active ones. The failure to repair potentially lethal lesions of DNA in active tissues virtually eliminates any chance for survival and therefore, effectively precludes the mutations from being expressed.

In addition to damaging DNA itself, irradiation can produce chromosomal damage which also is potentially lethal. Radiations can break chromosomes but unless cells carrying this injury attempt to divide, they seem to function normally. In this case, however, repair seems little influenced by the length of time after irradiation cell division occurs. Broken chromosomes can heal, but unless they do so within a few minutes of breakage, there is little further likelihood of healing.

At division, unhealed chromosome-breaks present an obstacle to proper distribution of genes to daughter cells and resulting imbalances often cause cell death (Fig. 7–1). Again, the degree of mitotic activity in tissue will affect that tissue's status after irradiation. Mitotically active tissues quickly purge themselves of cells which are chromosomally damaged, while static ones may retain this type of damage for a long time. Mitotically active tissues may suffer greater cell loss soon after irradiation than static ones, but the surviving population may be healthier.

Cellular reproductive mechanisms may also be damaged by irradiation. Precisely what structure or structures are injured is not known, but some authors believe nuclear membranes are involved. In any case, some irradiated cells immediately are rendered incapable of reproduction while others, though injured, can still reproduce. From the refer-

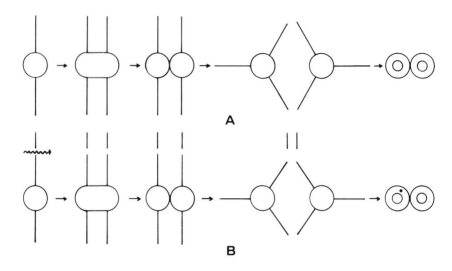

Fig. 7–1. *A mechanism for the production of imbalances in gene distribution during mitosis. A. Normal chromosome replication and distribution of genes. The chromosomal region of spindle attachment increases in size and the existing chromosomal thread directs the synthesis of an identical duplicate. The spindle attachment region cleaves, fibers attach, and identical chromosomes move away from each other to be incorporated in each daughter nucleus. B. Radiation breaks the chromosomal thread. Enlargement and cleavage of spindle attachment region occurs normally as does thread duplication. Fibers attach but the fragments are not drawn into daughter nuclei. Instead, they form a micronucleus in the cytoplasm of one of the two daughter cells. That daughter receives too many genes, the other too few.*

ence point of non-surgical cancer therapy, continued reproductive capacity after irradiation is undesirable. Proliferation of irradiated cancer cells presents a hazard to the patient. It means his or her cancer will be capable of further growth and spread. Furthermore, it appears that cells with sublethally injured reproductive mechanisms repair their injuries and eventually become indistinguishable in that regard, from cells which never were damaged. Consequently, if irradiation does not end but only injures cellular proliferative capacity, it may be fully repaired, in relatively short time periods. The production of irreparable damage to the reproductive ability of cancer cells, therefore, is clearly a desirable goal.

Relatively Effective Radiations. Cellular injury is produced when radiations dissipate their energy in cellular nuclei by ionization of molecules they find there. The patterns of energy dissipation by ionization differ for various radiations. As they traverse cellular matter, some

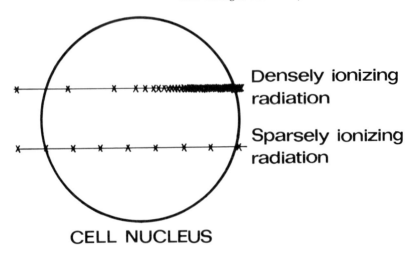

Fig. 7–2.   *Drawing depicting the path of two ionizing radiations through a cell nucleus. The densely ionizing one dissipates much energy per unit of its path (particularly at its end) in the form of many ionizations packed closely together. The sparsely ionizing radiation dissipates little energy in the same space and the ionizations it causes are few and far between.*

leave a dense track of ionization behind them and others, a sparse track (Fig. 7–2).

Densely ionizing radiations are more *effective* at producing cellular injuries than are sparsely ionizing radiations. Relatively small amounts of densely ionizing radiations produce the same level of damage as much greater amounts of sparsely ionizing radiations. Very densely ionizing radiations are so effective at producing injury that if one passes through a cell nucleus, the odds are overwhelming that it will kill that cell. Speaking practically, these radiations sterilize every cell through which they pass.

Sparsely ionizing radiations produce the opposite effect. Ionizations occur so infrequently as these radiations pass through cells, that the likelihood of any given radiation killing a cell is quite small. The cellular injuries produced are usually *sub*lethal. To achieve cell sterilization with sparsely ionizing rays, relatively large numbers of radiations must pass through cell nuclei. When that happens, the ion density produced by the many radiations will be high, equivalent to that of a densely ionizing radiation and therefore, likely to be lethal (Fig. 7–3).

The kinds of radiations in common use in radiotherapy today are sparsely ionizing, but the considerations mentioned above suggest that densely ionizing radiations ought to be much more effective at cancer

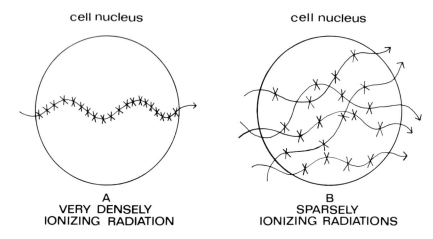

Fig. 7–3. *Comparison of the effects of very densely and sparsely ionizing radiations. A. A very densely ionizing radiation passes through a cell nucleus and produces 20 ionizations that (in this example) kill the cell. This single radiation is lethal; no sublethal effect or damage is registered. B. Five sparsely ionizing radiations traverse a cell nucleus. Each produces few ionizations and alone is not lethal. The five radiations together produce 20 ionizations and the cell dies. The densely ionizing radiation is relatively more effective than the sparsely ionizing ones by a factor of 5.*

cell sterilization. Trials are now underway to determine whether they meet their theoretical promise, but it is too early to make judgments. Unless they prove to be remarkably superior to conventional radiations, several imposing obstacles stand in the way of widespread clinical usage. While sparsely ionizing radiations (X and gamma rays) are relatively easily and cheaply obtained, densely ionizing radiations are not. Densely ionizing radiations suitable for medical use can only be generated by sources so large and expensive (as compared to those necessary for sparsely ionizing radiations) that even if clinically usable, they will be limited to a few large centers. Consequently, their clinical superiority will have to be convincingly shown before they will achieve wide acceptance.

Dose Equivalence. The likelihood of *cell* killing by commonly available, current methods, can be viewed as a kind of race between the rate of repair of sublethal damage and the rate of induction of damage (both lethal and sublethal) within every irradiated cell. *Tissue* damage depends upon the number of cells being irradiated and for this reason volume of treatment also acquires significance but, at the most basic level, the rates of damage and repair within each cell determine outcome. Three important concepts can be explained on this basis: (1) The tumoricidal effect of treatment at one anatomic site has *NO DIRECT IMPACT* on its tumoricidal effect at another site. In other words, doses of radiation delivered to more than one site *CANNOT BE ADDED* to arrive at a "total dose," (2) treatment given to the same anatomic site must be described in terms of energy absorbed from a specific number of fractions within a specific time frame, e.g., 5000 rad in 25 fractions over 35 days, and (3) the numerical descriptions of two courses of therapy given to the same site at different times cannot be added to produce a "total dose". Although several complex systems designed to calculate equivalent doses by compensating for repair between courses of treatment have been offered, none is precisely accurate and the concept of equivalent doses remains only loosely defined.

Chemotherapy. The effect of chemotherapeutic drugs may not be too different from that of ionizing radiation. As with sparsely ionizing radiations, their effects in cells are not all-or-nothing, but various levels of damage can result from their use. Further, it also appears that sublethal forms of damage they cause are reparable.[1]

Chemotherapeutic Targets. As is well known, the essence of living matter is embodied in three complex chemicals: DNA, RNA and protein. DNA is the basic blueprint of life and RNA translates this blueprint into the structural and functional unit of life, protein. Consequently, any drug that substantially interferes with normal synthesis of DNA, RNA or protein, or can disrupt already synthesized DNA, RNA or protein, can retard cell growth and perhaps cause death. When a drug is preferentially active in one or more of these ways against tumor cells, it qualifies for chemotherapeutic use.

Some chemotherapeutic agents act to inhibit the synthesis of DNA; others destroy already formed DNA; others block production of RNA while still others destroy specific proteins (Fig. 7–4).

Sites of Action. DNA is composed of two interconnected chains of organic bases called purines and pyrimidines. Of the many purines and pyrimidines, only two purines—adenine and guanine—and two pyrimidines—cytosine and thymine—occur in DNA (RNA is very similar, although it has only one chain and the base uracil replaces thymine). Before purine or pyrimidine bases can become part of DNA or RNA, they must be assembled from smaller molecules and many

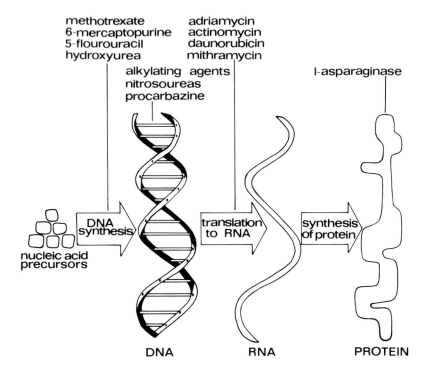

Fig. 7–4. *Schematic representation of sites of chemotherapeutic action on DNA to RNA to protein sequence.*

chemotherapeutic agents act to inhibit their synthesis. Methotrexate, 6-mercaptopurine, 6-thioguanine, 5-fluorouracil, cytosine arabinoside, and hydroxyurea all function, at least in part, in this manner. In addition, cytosine arabinoside inhibits the enzyme DNA polymerase which is instrumental in assembling the DNA chain.

Other drugs act upon already formed DNA. Nitrogen mustard, chlorambucil (leukeran), L-phenylalanine mustard (melphalan, L-PAM), and cyclophosphamide (cytoxan) all act in this manner by producing abnormal bonds in the DNA chain, disrupting its structure and function. The effect is so similar to that produced by radiation that these drugs are described as "radiomimetic." The nitrosoureas, BCNU and CCNU, appear to act in a similar fashion, distorting the structure of DNA. Procarbazine functions by literally hydrolyzing the normally connected DNA chains apart.

Drugs which prevent the functioning of DNA by interfering with its ability to direct RNA synthesis, in effect, produce the same practical

Table 7–1.   Classification and Mode of Action of Common
              Chemotherapeutic Agents

Alkylating Agents (attack formed DNA chains)
Nitrogen mustard
Chlorambucil (leukeran)
Cyclophosphamide (cytoxan)
L-phenylalanine mustard (L-PAM, melphalan)
Busulfan

Antimetabolites (block DNA synthesis)
Methotrexate
6-Mercaptopurine
5-Fluorouracil
Cytosine arabinoside
Thioguanine

Antibiotics (interfere with RNA synthesis)
Doxorubicin (adriamycin)
Bleomycin
Actinomycin-D
Mitomycin

Plant Alkaloids (interfere with spindle formation)
Vincristine (oncovin)
Vinblastine (velban)

results as drugs which alter its structure. In either case, RNA cannot be produced accurately. Adriamycin, actinomycin-D and mithramycin have this mode of action. The reader should not be fooled into thinking that drugs which only *interfere* with DNA function are less toxic than those which destroy its structure. Adriamycin and actinomycin, particularly in patients who also have received radiation, are two of the most, if not *the* most, toxic drugs in common use. Table 7–1 summarizes the classification of common antineoplastic drugs.

One additional way in which the DNA, RNA, protein synthesis sequence can be interrupted is by destroying proteins as they are made. In practice, this usually is not feasible because cells merely synthesize more and more protein until their needs are met; however, some neoplastic cells cannot produce certain proteins, such as asparagine, which are essential for their survival. These cells must rely upon a constant supply of asparagine from surrounding normal cells. The drug L-asparaginase hydrolyzes circulating asparagine and thereby starves dependent tumor cells.

Combination Radiation and Chemotherapy. The effects of radiation and drugs on cancers make each a good adjunct to the other in cancer therapy. For example, when various drugs are given, substantial sub-lethal damage may be inflicted upon cells of a cancer, but normal cells of other tissues of the body also will be affected. Tolerance of normal tissues consequently limits the dose that can be used against tumor. However, the *local* nature of radiotherapy permits additional injury to be added to the tumor while sparing the remainder of the body.

This methodology is, within limits, successful, and combinations of chemotherapy and radiation therapy are being used increasingly in non-surgical oncology.

Often several drugs are used together with irradiation. However, this technique usually is reserved for cases where it is felt that either method alone is likely to fail, because the total toxicity of treatment usually increases along with its efficacy as will be described in subsequent chapters.

Reference

1. Cole, W.H.: Chemotherapy of Cancer. Lea & Febiger. Philadelphia, 1970, p. 57.

8

EFFECT OF CELL
KINETICS

The effect of anticancer agents upon cells is not constant but changes at various times. Certain times, or phases, in cells' lifespans characteristically exhibit greater or lesser sensitivity to radiation and/or chemotherapeutic agents. A discussion of these phases and their influence upon the manner in which oncology is practiced form the subject of this chapter.

Cell Life Cycle. All cells arise from pre-existing cells. At some point in the life of a cell, it will begin to reproduce and, when reproduction is complete, it will have been replaced by two daughters. The daughters then mature and at some point in *their* lives may also reproduce. Clearly, cellular life consists of cycles, reproductive phases alternating with periods called *interphases*. During interphase, cells are functional, synthesizing protein and/or performing various functions for themselves and the organism of which they are a part. During reproductive phases, cells multiply, each cell undergoing division and producing two.

The length of interphase varies greatly. In rapidly proliferating cell populations (testis; bone marrow; mucosal lining of the small intestine) it is characteristically short, but in slowly proliferating populations (muscle, nerve) it is quite long. The length of the reproductive period, however, is fairly constant for all types of mammalian cells.

The reproductive phase can be divided into three subphases during which different processes presumably occur (Fig. 8–1). The first subphase to have been identified is called "M", for mitosis. In the late 19th and early 20th centuries, stains were developed which color chromatin, the genetic matter. In M, chromatin condenses and aggregates,

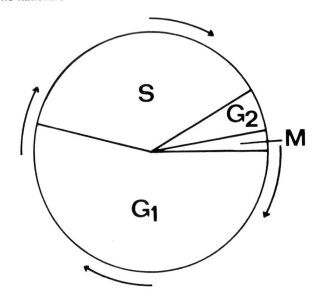

CELL LIFE CYCLE

Fig. 8–1. *Schematic representation of the life cycle of a cell. G_1 is the interphase, a stage preceding reproduction. The reproductive phases are called S, G_2 and M, respectively. The life cycle begins just as cells complete M and enter G_1, the interphase.*

forming structures called *chromosomes*. In a series of movements, the chromosomes replicate (prophase) and move from the equator of a reproducing cell (metaphase) to its poles (anaphase), giving rise to the two nuclei of the daughter cells (telophase).

The second phase to have been identified was "S", the time of DNA synthesis. In the 1950s radioactive precursors to DNA were made available and by radiographic techniques it became possible to recognize the time during which DNA was synthesized. Immediately, it also became obvious that, between M and S, there was an unaccounted-for time gap and, between S and M, there was another time gap. Since the processes occurring in these time gaps have not been identified, these periods have been called G_1 (gap 1) and G_2 (gap 2) respectively. G_1 is the *interphase* to which we have already referred. G_2 occurs *between* the synthesis of new DNA and mitosis. What happens during G_2 is not known for certain.

Radiation and the Cell Cycle. The position occupied by cells in the life cycle substantially influences the effect radiations have on their reproductive capacity. Generally G_1, the interphase, is a time of minimal responsiveness to irradiation. The reasons for this are not clear, but it is either a period of extraordinary radioresistance, a period in which cellular capacity for repair of radiation damage is high, or a period in which there is sufficient *time* for much radiation damage repair. Whatever is the case, cells irradiated in G_1 are not easily sterilized. If all else is equal, a cancer in which there are relatively few proliferating cells (a slow growing tumor or an old one) will be less radioresponsive than one in which many cells are proliferating.

Cells in proliferative stages of life cycle, S, G_2 and M (Fig. 8–1) are considerably more sensitive than those in G_1. However, when these stages are compared to each other, there are differences in the way their cells respond to irradiation. For example, it is a fair generalization to say that most cells, during much of S phase, are radioresistant when compared to G_2 and M, especially when using sparsely ionizing radiations such as X and gamma rays. The *degree* of radioresistance of S compared to G_2 and M varies among cells, but differences of factors of 2 or 3 are not uncommon. This means that, to sterilize cells in S—using X or gamma rays—a radiation dose 2 to 3 times greater than that required to produce the same endpoint in cells in G_2 or M will be needed. Densely ionizing radiations, on the other hand, will produce more uniform responses among the proliferative stages than sparsely ionizing rays and there may be little or no variation in response to *very* densely ionizing radiations.

Proliferative Delay. The variation in radiation response among proliferative phases is significant in establishing the condition of a cancer following irradiation. During irradiation, greatest damage (per unit of radiation dose) is done to cells in G_2 and M, while the least damage is done to those in S. After irradiation, radiation damaged cells stop progressing through the proliferative stages of the life cycle and are, for variable time periods, arrested in cycle. Teleologically speaking, the reason for this arrest is to give cells time to repair radiation damage. The length of arrest depends on various factors; size of the radiation dose, and phase of reproductive cycle in which radiation was delivered being two important ones. Large radiation doses produce longer delays than small ones, quite possibly because they cause more damage, requiring more time to repair. Delay following irradiation with any given dose is longer in sensitive phases than resistant ones so that cells in S usually are delayed less than those in G_2 or M. The result is that cells which are in S during irradiation begin to progress through

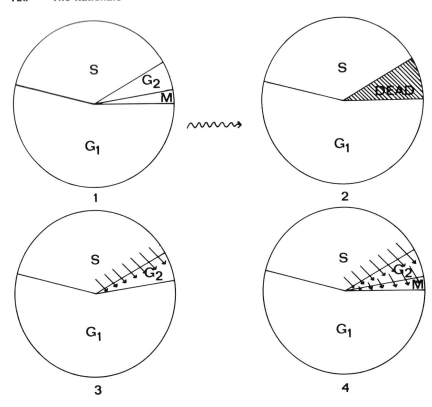

PRODUCTION OF SYNCHRONY

Fig. 8–2. *Mechanism of radiation induced synchrony. Normal cell cycle (1). Radiation prefer-entially kills cells in G_2 and M (2). The cohort of cells moves synchronously into G_2 (3) and subsequently into M (4).*

life cycle before those in G_2 and M. In this way, irradiation creates a more-or-less synchronously dividing population of cells; in the first hours post-irradiation only those cells in S *during irradiation* have recovered and are moving through reproductive phases (Fig. 8–2). This is important in two ways. *First*, this cohort of cells moves from S to G_2 and M, phases which are quite radiosensitive. If the exact time required for synchronously dividing cells to reach these phases could be determined, then a second dose of radiation could be given at that time. Presumably this second radiation dose would find a cell population all in the same sensitive phase and would be efficient at cell killing. Unfortunately, it is not now possible to accomplish this at the clinical level, but it is an area of research and a method which may be in the future of non-surgical oncology.

The *second* way in which radiation-produced synchrony is important will be described in greater detail later in this chapter. By establishing a cell population proceeding simultaneously through life cycle, phase-specific chemotherapeutic agents can be used more effectively and successfully. Radiation can establish synchrony and drugs can be applied when many cells are in the phase most sensitive to them.

Cell Generation Time. In light of the marked differences in sensitivity to irradiation during different phases of life cycle, it should be obvious that radiosensitivity of a cancer or tissue depends on how many of its cells are in mitosis, how often they reproduce. Among tissues and cancers, interphase (G_1) varies greatly in length, so that the

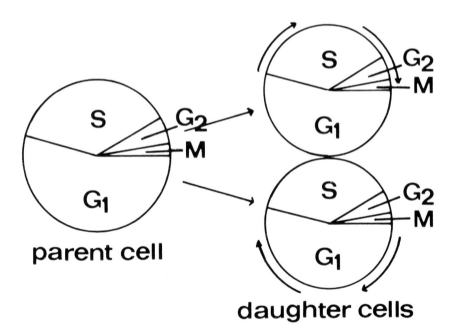

GENERATION TIME

Fig. 8–3.   *An illustration of cell generation time. The parent cell has reproduced to yield two daughter cells. The daughters are now reproducing, each to produce two daughters of their own. The time elapsed between the same stage in parental and daughter life cycles is called generation time. For example, the number of hours, days, weeks or years between S in the parental cycle and S in the daughters' cycle is the generation time.*

time taken for one cycle varies. The time required for one complete cycle, the cell generation time (Fig. 8–3), varies considerably and forms a characteristic of the cell which has relevance in nonsurgical oncology.

In tissues in which many cells are produced, generation time is short, measured in hours to a few days. In tissues in which few cells are being produced, generation time is long, measured in weeks to months and perhaps years.

In response to extraordinary conditions, generation time can change. When a tissue has been injured and there has been substantial loss of cells, remaining cells respond by attempting to replenish the cell population quickly. One way in which this is accomplished is by *shortening* generation time in surviving cells. This enables a greater number of cells to be produced in any given time interval. Once the cell population is restored to normal numbers, generation time reverts to its usual interval.

Irradiation, of course, is an agent which depletes cell populations; in sufficient dosage it kills and injures relatively large numbers of proliferating cells. In normal tissues, remaining proliferative cells (presumably uninjured or repaired cells) respond to the emergency caused by irradiation by shortening generation time in an attempt to repopulate the tissue. Any lapse in tissue function is kept to short periods this way.

Cancer cells do not respond the same way. Quite possibly because they are not fully under control of host homeostatic mechanisms which are believed to direct repopulation of tissues after substantial cell loss, cell generation time of cancer cells either does not change after irradiation, or sometimes even lengthens. After injury by irradiation, cancers do not attempt to repopulate themselves in the same way as normal tissues. Consequently, after irradiation an advantage would seem to go to normal tissues. They act quickly to restore cell number while cancers do not. In competition for space, oxygen and nutrient, after radiation injury to normal tissues and cancers, normal tissues can repopulate quickly filling space and taking oxygen and nutrient. On these grounds alone, irradiation should be so advantageous to normal tissue that irradiated cancers would be reduced in size, possibly enough to disappear altogether.

Cells in G_0. But there are other reasons favoring normal tissues over cancers. Within the G_1 population of normal tissue is a subpopulation of cells which seems to *retain* proliferative capacity, although under usual circumstances does not proliferate. These cells have been designated as being in a life phase called G_0. When there is a sudden demand for cells, such as occurs when a tissue is injured and many cells are lost, G_0 cells quickly enter proliferative cycle. The entry of these cells into cycle adds to the number already proliferating and makes possible the production of many new cells. G_0 cells, therefore, seem to constitute a reserve, giving tissues the ability to respond to serious cell loss.

So far, no analogous situation has been detected in cancers. Consequently, after irradiation, which reduces their cell population, no reserve seems to exist enabling them to repopulate rapidly.

In summary, cancers, lacking a G_0 population and the capacity to shorten generation time, seem not as well equipped to *repopulate* following irradiation as normal tissue. Escape from homeostasis appears a mixed blessing. On one hand, cancers are free to do what normal tissues may not; invade, metastasize and subvert metabolism. On the other, they cannot respond well to injury such as is produced by irradiation. The net advantage, at least for individual lesions, seems to fall to normal tissues.

Chemotherapy. When compared to the influence of cell type on the clinical choice of drug for cancer therapy, the influence of cell kinetics is minor. To date, the decision to use a specific drug for a specific tumor, has been made almost entirely on the basis of prior clinical experience. The drug that has produced a beneficial response most frequently has become the drug of choice; less effective agents are used only when first-line therapy fails. Crude as this system may be, it is effective.

Nevertheless, theoretical considerations suggest that kinetics should not be irrelevant in chemotherapeutic management. A study of interactions between drugs and cycling cells may well lead to better understanding and more intelligent use of drugs in hand, as well as the development of new ones. Already, it permits identification of drugs with similar mechanisms of action, which to some degree, has been and almost surely will continue to be a substantial aid in design of effective programs using combinations of drugs and treatment schedules which exploit cellular kinetics.

Cell Cycle. Because various anti-neoplastic agents have different mechanisms of action, they exert different degrees of influence at different times in cell cycle.[1] Drugs that inhibit synthesis of DNA *precursors* produce their greatest effects when cells are in the S phase, trying to synthesize DNA. However, the action of all drugs is not affected by cell cycle to the same degree. The marked similarity in structure of RNA and DNA results in their need for several common precursors. Some drugs which inhibit DNA precursor synthesis also inhibit the formation of RNA precursors. Because RNA is critical to protein synthesis, lack of RNA inhibits protein formation. Lack of protein slows down metabolism and, in fact, the entire cell cycle. When the cycle is slower the chance that a cell will progress *into* the highly sensitive S phase is reduced. By reducing the number of cells entering S, the poisons that *also* inhibit RNA actually are somewhat self-defeating. Drugs which specifically inhibit only DNA synthesis, e.g., cytosine arabinoside or hydroxyurea, are more S phase dependent than those which inhibit both RNA and DNA synthesis; e.g., methotrexate or 5-fluorouracil.

In contrast, vincristine and vinblastine preferentially are effective in the M phase of cell cycle. In tissue culture, they can be seen to destroy spindle fibers which normally act to separate chromosomes during mitosis. Consequently, cell cycle abruptly stops in metaphase (metaphase arrest).

Drugs which interfere with structure and function of already synthesized DNA exert their effects independent of cell cycle (e.g., alkylating agents).

Effect of Cell Cycle on Combination Chemotherapy. When single agents are selected for use against various cancers, kinetic considerations usually are ignored and agents are picked on the basis of expected response rates. However, every agent has inherent limitations. We are beginning to learn that drugs sometimes must be combined to achieve maximum benefit. But what combinations are likely to be most effective?

Combination chemotherapy, like single agent therapy, could be developed empirically. However, this route would be tedious, inefficient and would sacrifice many lives. *First*, the optimum number of drugs for treatment of every individual type of tumor would have to be determined. *Second*, assuming that this could be done, and for the sake of argument, 3-drug combinations were found optimal, from the available pool of approximately 70 active drugs, nearly 50,000 combinations of 3-drugs would have to be tested.[2] *Third*, optimum dose levels of *each* drug would have to be determined. Because of toxicity of each drug, it would be virtually impossible to design a combination that utilized each at the maximum level permissable when the drug is used alone; rather, each drug would probably have to be used at a fraction of this dose, prompting the need for huge studies. For example, to determine the optimum dose level for each of a 5-drug *combination* requires 32 trials if only 2 levels are tested, and 243 trials if 3 levels are considered.[2] *Fourth*, the optimum timing of each drug within the combination would have to be determined, and this would add further to the complexity of such a search.

The ability to predict *beforehand* which combination drug regimens have a greater than average chance of being successful would avoid so long and costly a search and, unquestionably, would be distinctly helpful. The manner in which each chemotherapeutic agent produces its effects forms one basis by which combinations can be designed. Agents which act through the same, or similar, mechanisms are likely to produce little more than increased doses of either one when added together. In contrast, the combination of two *dissimilar* agents may be more effective than either agent, at any dose level.

The validity of this concept can be shown by examining drug combinations of demonstrated efficacy. Consider the combination of nitrogen mustard, oncovin (vincristine), procarbazine and prednisone (MOPP) which has proven of value in the treatment of Hodgkin's disease. Nitrogen mustard is an alkylating agent acting to form abnormal linkages in DNA; vincristine is a mitotic spindle poison; procarbazine hydrolyzes DNA and prednisone, a steroid, probably acts to alter the rate of protein synthesis. Similarly, the combination of cyclophosphamide (cytoxan), vincristine and prednisone (COP or CVP), used for lymphocytic lymphomas follows the same basic format, in this case the alkylating agent, cyclophosphamide, substitutes for the alkylating agent, nitrogen mustard. And when this combination is expanded by the addition of adriamycin (CHOP) for the non-lymphocytic lymphomas, it is more than coincidental that the additional agent acts in a unique fashion; i.e., by inhibiting translation of DNA into RNA. Last, consider the combination of cyclophosphamide, methotrexate, and 5-fluorouracil (CMF), described in Chapter 5 for use against breast cancer. The combination joins an alkylating agent with two antimetabolites, each of which inhibits the formation of DNA precursors, but by different mechanisms. And, in the expanded versions of this combination which includes vincristine and prednisone (CMFVP), note that the additional agents each act in a different manner from any of the other drugs.

Phase Specificity. Just as classification can aid in selection of drugs, examination of kinetic data can provide a rational basis for timing of chemotherapy. Bruce et al.[3] considered the differential action of various drugs at different dose levels on neoplastic (lymphoma) cells and normal hematopoietic stem cells. They found that three different types of responses occur. Some drugs, e.g., nitrogen mustard, kill malignant and normal cells in culture equally and are, therefore, termed *nonspecific*. A second class of drugs, e.g., vinblastine, preferentially kills neoplastic cells; however, once a specific dose level is reached, no further killing takes place. The authors deduced that only a proportion of the exposed cells were sensitive to these agents and that these cells were sensitive because they were in a specific *phase* of the cycle. Such drugs are, therefore, termed *phase-specific*. The third class of drugs, e.g., actinomycin-D, produce preferential killing of tumor cells but do not have a dose dependent maximum effect. It appears that this response occurs because of greater proliferative activity of tumor cells than normal cells. Consequently, these drugs are believed to act only upon growing cells, i.e., those cells in cycle. Because they do not appear to depend upon a particular phase of the cycle but rather are active throughout, such drugs are termed *cycle*-specific.

This classification system carries predictive value for optimal timing of chemotherapy. In theory, cycle-specific agents should be given infrequently and at maximum tolerable doses[4] to avoid normal cells, which mainly are not in cycle, while killing malignant cells, which are. Repetitive doses would draw normal cells into cycle, thereby decreasing the therapeutic effectiveness of the drug. In contrast, phase-specific drugs need to be given either repetitively or be constantly infused to insure that all tumor cells are exposed to the drug as they pass through sensitive phases of cycle. Unfortunately, in practice, the length of treatment is limited by entry of normal cells into cycle. The drug must be discontinued before many normal cells reach the deadly phase.

Some clinical data exist to support these hypotheses. For example, cytosine arabinoside, a phase specific drug, preferentially is administered by repetitive doses or infusion.[5] Similarly, the efficacy of vinblastine, when given as a continuous infusion, can be explained on this basis.

Synchronization. One of the limitations of clinical chemotherapeutic management is imposed by asynchrony of cells within a tumor. While some cells are in sensitive phases, others are insensitive. As a result, only some tumor cells are killed.

A solution to this problem, at least in theory, would result if all tumor cells could be synchronized in a sensitive phase. A number of procedures which will synchronize cells in *tissue culture* can be found in the literature.[6] However, technical difficulties currently preclude the translation of these experimental procedures into routine clinical practice.

Cell Compartments. Kinetic data also explain failure of chemotherapy on other bases. As already has been discussed, in cancers some cells are actively proliferating; others are *capable* of division but at a given time are not dividing, and some cells appear incapable of division. As in the case described for irradiation, quiescent but *potentially* clonogenic cells create the major obstacle to successful chemotherapy. Actively dividing cells are preferentially killed by either phase-specific or cycle-specific agents and permanently non-dividing cells, because of their very nature, cannot multiply and threaten a patient's life. On the other hand, potentially clonogenic cells are protected from the action of most drugs when they are out of cell cycle but can enter cycle and reproduce once drug is terminated. Thus, such cells account for one mechanism of failure of chemotherapy.

Recruitment. Recruitment is to cycle-specificity as synchronization is to phase-specificity. In essence, recruitment is a strategy which initially employs a drug acting relatively independent of cell cycle. The resulting tumor cell destruction tends to draw non-proliferating tumor cells into cycle. The precise reasons for entry of quiescent tumor cells into cycle are not clear, but a fair assumption is that death of proliferative cells improves oxygen and nutrient supply for the rest. The improvement permits proliferation. At this point, highly cycle- or phase-specific drugs are administered and produce a greater anti-tumor effect than if they had been used initially. In vitro models validate the logic of this approach. For example, recruitment of tumor cells by the drug cyclophosphamide permits cytosine arabinoside to destroy an experimental plasmacytoma which previously had been insensitive.[7]

Resistance to Drugs. Tumor cells also may be insensitive to a specific drug or drugs for other reasons. Hall[8] notes that there are three different types of resistance: innate, acquired and collateral.

Tumors which have *innate* resistance withstand the action of a chemotherapeutic agent the first time they come into contact with the drug. Whatever affords the tumor its protection is inherent in its nature, prior to its exposure to the drug.

Tumors which *acquire* resistance initially are susceptible to the drug. However, during the period of sensitivity, the tumor adapts and eventually manages to circumvent the drug's action. When this occurs, the tumor begins to grow anew and the patient goes into clinical relapse.

Uncommonly, resistance to a drug is evoked by the presence of a second drug. The effect of the second drug brings about a change in the tumor which shields it from damage done by the first drug. Because of the crucial role of the second drug in this process, this type of change is called *collateral* resistance.

Mechanisms of Resistance. Although classification into innate, acquired and collateral resistance describes the fashion in which tumors escape chemotherapeutic control, it does not describe a mechanism by which this happens and it is known that many varied *mechanisms* of resistance are possible. For example, Hall[8] lists ten different cellular adaptations which can account for a tumor's ability to resist damage, including altered pathways of DNA synthesis, increased DNA synthesis, and increased capacity to repair drug induced damage. In many instances, more than one mechanism operates simultaneously.

The principal mechanism or mechanisms of resistance in a given case, to some extent, reflect the chemotherapeutic agent being used. Alkylating agents tend to increase the capacity to repair DNA; antibiotic chemotherapeutic agents do not appear to be retained within some tumor cells; antimetabolites are not transported into target cells; hormonal agents are not transported into the nucleus where they are active when specific receptor proteins are not present in the tumor's cytoplasm. Thus, the primary mechanisms by which tumors escape chemotherapeutic control are not totally unknown. The implication that it may be possible to understand the precise mechanisms in a given case sufficiently well to permit design of programs of therapy which will circumvent or perhaps even exploit these mechanisms, is inescapable.

Prediction of Response. In vitro data also may provide a basis for prediction of response or lack of response prior to therapy. In theory, such data would permit selection of drugs for therapy which have a better chance of success than others. It is even possible, in given cases, that the combination with the best chance of success could be chosen. At present, attempts to use data in this manner for clinical purposes have been limited by technical considerations. To succeed, a specific test predicting response or lack of response would have to be available.

In addition, a relatively "pure" source of tumor cells would be required, and if a number of determinations need to be done, the source must be able to yield large numbers of cells.

For some types of tumors these requirements can be met. Leukemias easily can be sampled and tests are available which will, at least, predict lack of response to certain drugs. If leukemic cells, incubated with radiolabeled methotrexate do not retain the drug, tumor response is unlikely.[9] Similar analysis will identify leukemias which will not respond to 6-mercaptopurine or cytosine arabinoside.[10,11] Although such analysis is too complex for routine clinical use at present and is not yet applicable for the vast majority of cancers, it suggests another direction for future progress.

Accessory Agents. In vitro data provide yet another basis for chemotherapeutic management. Although selection of single agents by trial and error is feasible, for the many reasons already discussed, empiric methods are an inefficient way to design combinations of drugs. As a result, combinations nearly always are designed by adding together drugs which are effective individually. And yet, there are situations in which agents which are ineffective by themselves, substantially improve the efficacy of another agent or agents. In vitro data can help predict when this will happen.

In most cases, accessory agents act to ameliorate the toxicity of the effective agent, thereby permitting its more aggressive administration. For example, the maximum permissible dose of adriamycin is limited by cardiac toxicity. In mice[12] this effect is prevented by administration of vitamin E. It remains to be seen if the same relationship exists in man.

There already is one well known example of this principle in clinical practice. The drug methotrexate can be administered in seemingly prohibitive amounts if the toxic effects are subsequently ameliorated by administration of folinic acid to "rescue" normal cells (Chap. 11).

References

1. Krakoff, I.H.: Cancer Chemotherapeutic Agents. Ca—A Cancer Journal for Clinicians 23:208–219, 1973.
2. Lloyd, H.H.: Combination Chemotherapy: Considerations for Design and Analysis. Cancer Chemother. Rep. 4:157–165, 1974.
3. Bruce, W.R., Meeker, B.E., and Valeriote, F.A.: Comparison of the Sensitivity of Normal Hematopoietic and Transplanted Lymphoma Colony-Forming Cells to Chemotherapeutic Agents Administered in Vivo. J. Nat. Canc. Inst. 37:233–245, 1966.
4. Valeriote, F.A., and Edelstein, M.B.: The Role of Cell Kinetics in Cancer Chemotherapy. Semin. Oncol. 4:217–226, 1977.

5. Ho, *et al.*: In Sartorelli and Johns (eds.) *Antineoplastic and Immunosuppressive Agents*, Vol. 38/2, New York, Springer-Verlag, 1975, p. 257.
6. Nias, A.H.W., and Fox, M.: Synchronization of Mammalian Cells with Respect to the Mitotic Cycle. Cell Tissue Kinet. *4*:375–398, 1971.
7. Schabel, F.M., Jr.: The Use of Tumor Growth Kinetics in Planning "Curative" Chemotherapy of Advanced Solid Tumors. Cancer Res. *29*:2384–2389, 1969.
8. Hall, T.C.: Prediction of Responses to Therapy and Mechanisms of Resistance. Semin. Oncol. *4*:193–202, 1977.
9. Kessel, D., Hall, T.C., Roberts, D., and Wodinsky, I.: Uptake as a Determinant of Methotrexate Response In Mouse Leukemias. Science *150*:752–754, 1967.
10. Kessel, D., and Hall, T.C.: Retention of 6-mercaptopurine by Intact Cells as an Index of Drug Responsiveness in Human and Murine leukemias. Cancer Res. *29*:2116–2119, 1969.
11. ———: Transport and Phosphorylation as Factors in the Antitumor Action of Cytosine Arabinoside. Science *156*:1240–1241, 1967.
12. Myers, C.E., McGuire, W., and Young R.: Adriamycin: Amelioration of Toxicity by Alpha-Tocopherol. Cancer Treat. Rep. *60*:961–962, 1976.

THE
RATIONALE

Tissue
Level

9

Patterns of Cancer Growth

It is often said that cancers grow in a chaotic manner, implying that no pattern or organization to their growth exists. An image is conjured of rapid mitotic rates and rampant, formless growth, beyond host control, indeed, beyond any control at all. In recent years that picture has been modified, and it is recognized now that, while the manner of cancer growth significantly differs from that of normal tissue, there frequently can be perceived a growth pattern reminiscent of the tissue of origin—or at least of the embryonic germ layer from which both the normal tissue and cancer is derived. And, to some degree this pattern of growth often directly impinges on the ability to control them by non-surgical measures.

Normal Tissue. A comparison of growth patterns of normal tissues and cancers can be instructive. Normal tissues in different organs and at different times (presumably in response to homeostatic genetic control) can exhibit differing growth patterns. Embryonic life is characterized by high mitotic rates. All early embryonic cells appear to be proliferative, each dividing cell giving rise to daughter cells capable of replication. In time, however, this pattern changes and a proportion of embryonic cells becomes non-proliferative; these cells specialize and carry out specific tissue functions for the organism and, presumably, are unable to divide. Others are quiescent, but they can become proliferative if the organism's needs demand it.

From nearly all normal tissues, cell loss occurs. Fully differentiated, specialized, functional cells cannot reproduce, and at the end of their life spans, (which in most instances are not as long as the life of the organism) must be replaced by descendants of proliferative cells in the tissue, which can differentiate and specialize in the tissue's function. During growth of the organism (childhood, adolescence and young adulthood), the number of cells produced by proliferative cells in tissues exceeds cell loss, and the tissue grows at a rate regulated by the organism's genes. During adulthood, in most tissues, the number of cells produced equals that lost and no further growth occurs. Equilibrium is established; there is no *net* cell gain or loss.

Some exceptions to this generalization occur. For example, as mature ova are shed from ovaries, they are not replaced and their number declines. Evidence exists suggesting that in *mature* central nervous tissue the life of functional cells equals that of the organism so that replacement is unnecessary. But these are exceptions; in general, in adults, cell loss equals cell gain.

Cancers. In cancers the situation is similar yet different. So far as experimental evidence can determine, cancers, too, begin as one or a few cells, all of which proliferate. Although they replicate and their daughters replicate, a point is reached at which some cells become quiescent (non-proliferative). In certain animal tumors in which this phenomenon has been studied, evidence suggests that a quiescent cell population comes into existence even when the cancer is extremely small, at or even beneath the limits of clinical detection. In part, this population becomes quiescent not because it has differentiated, but apparently because some of its cells have become hypoxic.

Growing cancers, like *growing* normal tissues, produce more cells than they lose. But in normal tissue, growth is regulated so that supporting vascular stroma grows and keeps pace with expanding cell number. In cancers this does not seem to be true. In growing normal tissue, all cells presumably have access to adequate nourishment and oxygen, but because vascular stroma supplying cancers fails to keep pace with cancer growth, a proportion of cancer cells becomes hypoxic and probably malnourished as well. Lack of adequate oxygen prevents hypoxic cells from proliferating, and they become quiescent. Should such cells regain access to oxygen, it is believed they can again become proliferative. Such cells are quiescent, then, not because they have come under some homeostatic restraint of either host or cancer, but because they lack the wherewithal with which to proliferate.

Another population of cells seems to exist in cancers. Some cells of cancers may not wholly escape host homeostatic control. The proliferative capacity of these cells is checked, not because of nutritional or oxygen deficit, but because the host controls them in much the same way as normal cell proliferation is controlled.

Finally, another category of quiescent cells has been suggested to exist in cancers. Some cancer cells may cease proliferating for unknown reasons and differentiate, exercising some or all of the functions of normal cells in the tissue of origin. This certainly indicates that there are cells in and of cancers in which malignant transformation is incomplete or weak. Such cells may become non-proliferative and even differentiate to function more-or-less normally.

Cancer, A Complex Structure. It must be clear from the foregoing that cancers are not simple, aggressive masses of fully proliferative cells, but fairly complex structures including a number of elements of normal tissue. A proliferating compartment can be recognized; there is a quiescent compartment; there are cells independent of host homeostasis, replicating *ad libidum*, and cells independent of homeostasis, quiescent because of oxygen and nutrient deficit; there may be quiescent cells subject to host homeostasis which are undifferentiated or non-functional and cells subject to homeostasis either partly or fully differentiated and functional. And it may be that when all is said and done, other cell types not now suspected may be found to exist.

Cell Loss Factor. As in normal tissue, cells are lost from cancers. As cancers age, the number of cells produced by the proliferating compartment (or *growth fraction*) lessens. The quiescent fraction of the cancer grows larger. Cells of the cancer, principally though not exclusively from the quiescent fraction, die, and this has become known as the "cell loss factor." Cell loss seems due to several factors: In those rapidly proliferating portions of cancers, cells, too far from capillaries, become progressively more hypoxic, ultimately to be anoxic and, without oxygen, die. Other cells may die because of host immunologic reaction against them; some quiescent cells under homeostatic restraint or cells which have differentiated, probably die simply because their life span is exhausted. Recently, evidence has come to light demonstrating cancer cell loss through a process termed "apoptosis." Apoptosis is a phenomenon observed in normal structures and can be defined as planned or programmed cell death. For example, resorption of embryonic structures, which do not persist to adulthood, occurs by apoptosis. Among these are the gill slits of mammalian embryos, the webbing between fingers in human embryos and tails of frog and salamander larvae. During apoptosis, cells become densely condensed and die. They fragment and are phagocytized by neighboring cells which are usually of the same type as the cell that has died.

The occurrence of apoptosis in cancers may suggest a number of possibilities. (1) Perhaps it is merely the persistence of a normal process but which, in neoplasia, has no specific function (a "memory," let us say, of normal ancestry). (2) It may suggest a degree of internal organization on the part of cancers or (3) partly successful host efforts to destroy the growth.

Response to Therapy. Whatever the source(s) of cell loss factor, it can be important in patterns of cancer growth. Cell loss factor, as determined from animal models, is quite high for carcinomas but much lower for sarcomas. This suggests that cell *loss* from the tumor may determine the *rate* of increase in size of carcinomas, while this factor may be much less significant in increase in size of sarcomas. In carcinomas, the number of cells produced only slightly exceeds the number lost (about 70% of cells produced are lost). Consequently, the net increase in amount of *living* tumor is small as time passes, but there often accumulates a considerable mass of dead and dying cells. Typically these cancers are composed of thin rims of living tissue and large necrotic and dying centers (Fig. 9–1).

In sarcomas, the number of cells lost is quite small compared to the number produced (about 30% of cells produced are lost). Con-

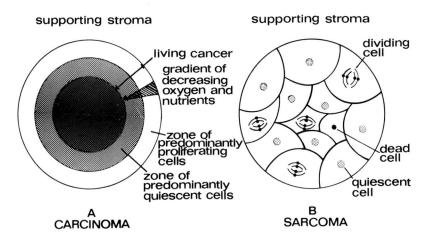

supporting stroma   supporting stroma

living cancer
gradient of decreasing oxygen and nutrients
dividing cell
zone of predominantly proliferating cells
zone of predominantly quiescent cells
dead cell
quiescent cell

A
CARCINOMA

B
SARCOMA

Fig. 9–1. *Schematic representation of structure of carcinomas and sarcomas.*

sequently, the net increase in amount of living tumor is great over time and there is little buildup of dead or dying tissue (Fig. 9–1).

Confusion may arise. Just because carcinomas lose many cells per unit of time does not mean they grow slowly. Just because sarcomas lose few cells with time does not mean they grow fast. The rate of growth of cancers also depends upon the *number* of cells dividing and the number of cells produced in given units of time. The *generation time* of cancer cells and the size of the growth fraction also influence growth rates (Chap. 8). These differences may explain, at least in part, the behavior of cancer types following irradiation. Irradiation affects *proliferating* cells most severely. Some are killed, some sterilized, others may be halted for varying lengths of time in progression through life cycle and the production of new cancer cells will be severely reduced (the degree of reduction due to a complex of factors including radiation dose). If cells continue to be lost at high rates after irradiation, as appears to be the case in carcinomas, they should shrink rapidly during and after treatment, a phenomenon frequently observed in the clinic.

It might be that the same number of *proliferating* cells in sarcomas would be killed during irradiation as in carcinomas, but, because so many fewer cells naturally are lost from sarcomas owing to their inherent pattern of growth, the tumors may well shrink much less rapidly.

Rapid regression of tumor during and just after therapy, does not necessarily insure a high probability of cure. Slow regression does not mean poor prognosis (Chap. 6). A carcinoma may regress dramatically during therapy owing to its intrinsic growth pattern, but regrowth may also occur, perhaps soon after treatment. Sarcomas may seem to respond hardly at all during therapy, but may shrink slowly over several weeks to months following therapy as its cells move slowly to death through the small cell loss factor. Overall, the number of "cures" may be much the same in both classes of cancer, even though the short term responses differ dramatically.

Effect of Growth Pattern on Radiotherapy. The response of cancers to radiation therapy depends upon a number of growth pattern factors: (1) The size of the proliferating or growth fraction (the portion of a tumor most vulnerable to radiation in which the largest number of cells will be killed); (2) The size and composition of the quiescent fraction (the portion of a tumor containing its resistant cells but those which, if conditions warrant or permit, can begin proliferation); (3) The size of the cell loss factor (the larger this factor the more rapidly cells are lost from the tumor mass). Irradiation presumably removes most cells from the proliferating compartment. Cells continue to be lost because of cell loss factors (immunologic rejection, apoptosis, anoxia), and if the rate is high, the tumor will get smaller quickly.

Effect of Growth Pattern on Chemotherapy. Response to chemotherapy is probably very much controlled by the pattern of tumor growth, also. First, and most obvious, the discrepancy in growth rate between tumor and its blood supply, which makes portions of tumor hypoxic and nutritionally deprived, probably affects distribution of chemotherapeutic drugs through tumor. It seems likely that inadequately oxygenated and fed cells also receive less drug—or receive it later—than well-aerated and well-fed portions. The result should be a greater cell kill in well-vascularized tumor sections, the sections, which, in all likelihood, contain the proliferating cells. Chemotherapy as well as radiation therapy affects most drastically the proliferating compartment and to lesser degrees, the quiescent. Clearly, then, the *size* of the proliferating compartment quite significantly affects the chemoresponsiveness of cancers (as is the case with radiation response). Cancers with large proliferating compartments will, all other things being equal, respond more profoundly to drugs than those in which the compartment is small. Since proliferating compartments usually are large (relative to the total tumor) when tumors are young and rapidly doubling in size, early diagnosed tumors have a better chance of being cured by both drugs and radiation than those which are older and larger and in which a significant quiescent compartment has grown (Chap. 10).

Not only do "young" cancers have large proliferating compartments compared to "old" ones of the same kind, but various tumor types differ in this regard. For example, carcinomas generally have large proliferative compartments, compared to quiescent compartments, and sarcomas have much smaller proliferative versus quiescent compartments. This may reflect the germ layer of origin of the two general categories of cancers. As previously noted, carcinomas are formed from tissues derived from ectodermal and entodermal structures (skin, linings of glands, linings of segments of the gastrointestinal tract), while sarcomas are derived of mesodermal tissues (muscle, bone, soft tissues). Tissues derived from ectoderm and entoderm have generally a high cell loss. In the natural course of events, cells are continuously shed from skin, lost from the linings of various glands, the mucosa of mouth and rectum at quite high rates. Replacement occurs at equally high rates in order for these tissues to maintain continuous optimum function. This necessitates large proliferative compartments. On the other hand, tissues derived from mesoderm have little cell loss per unit of time. Their functional cells have long lives and need replacement infrequently. This permits small proliferative compartments. Cancers derived from these normal tissues seem to imitate the normal tissue of origin in this respect.

Just as the proliferative compartment of tumors is important in determining the outcome of either radio- or chemotherapy, so too is the quiescent compartment important, particularly in the outcome of chemotherapy. Quiescent cells retaining proliferative capacity (quite possibly because of nutritional deficit) are those *most* likely to be spared killing action of antineoplastic drugs. From the foregoing it is clear that there probably are two reasons: (1) Quiescent cells are not proliferating and, in consequence, somewhat resistant to many drugs; (2) Nutritionally deprived cells, quiescent on that account, are likely to have lesser quantities of drug inflicted upon them, than upon those near feeding capillaries. After treatment with antineoplastic drugs, well-fed proliferating cancer cells probably die, leaving nutrient and oxygen for deprived, quiescent cells. Those that can, begin proliferating and a recurrence begins.

Normal Tissue Tolerance. In cancer control by either radiation or chemotherapy, normal tissues of the body play a role that would be difficult to overestimate. The quantity of radiation or antineoplastic drug that can be given a cancer is limited by tolerance of normal tissue, both in the short and long run. Cells of normal tissues respond as do those of cancers to non-surgical oncologic methods. During therapy, normal tissues—in the irradiated field or exposed to antineoplastic drugs—having large proliferative compartments suffer a large loss of cells. Usually such tissues also have a large natural cell loss factor, and they can deplete quite rapidly. In the short run, cell depletion from certain normal tissues can threaten life, and this limits dose of therapeutic agent. In the long run it is a factor also, but one not so much appreciated until recently. Even tissues with small cell loss factors and small proliferative compartments undergo cell loss as a result of therapy. Cells are lost slowly from these tissues, and months or years later, cell depletion occurs. Tissue function can be impaired long after treatment, resulting in complications of therapy and providing a dose limiting factor.

10

EFFECT OF TUMOR
SIZE

The success of anticancer therapy depends greatly on tumor size. Larger tumors are both more difficult to control locally and more likely to give rise to distant metastases than are small ones of the same kind. To some extent, larger tumors imply either that they have been present for relatively prolonged periods of time (to attain their size) and represent late stage disease or that they are extremely rapidly growing, aggressive lesions which are, in effect, beyond host control. Any one of the above factors by itself influences prognosis adversely and combinations usually are evident in clinical practice. The purpose of this chapter, therefore, is to discuss the manner in which management is influenced by the size of a tumor and to look at methods which have been developed to cope with, and at times exploit, differences in tumor size.

Tumor Growth and Differentiation. Tumors, benign or malignant, probably begin from a single or a few genetically transformed cells. Initially, little need for competition among these cells exists, so that when cancers are young (microscopic size disease), most if not all of their cells are proliferative. However, early in the natural history of cancers as discussed in previous chapters, some cells begin to exhibit characteristics different from each other. Whether this constitutes true differentiation as occurs during embryogenesis or during the production of mature, functional cells from tissue stem cells, remains to be clarified. But, in any event, some cancer cells begin to differ from the rest and a few of them acquire or express the capacity to metastasize.[1] Somehow, these cells break through the walls of blood vessels and detach from the tumor mass. The process of breakthrough and detachment may well go on through much of the life of a cancer, but only a select few detached cells are able to survive long in the blood stream, which for non-hematogenous cells, is a hostile environment. Fewer yet eventually succeed in "taking" in some distant organ and begin the process of forming a new tumor, a metastasis. The sites of metastasis are evidently not a matter of pure chance, but the result of a particular propensity of specific cancer cells (Chap. 12). Experiments have shown that circulating tumor cells do not necessarily give rise to metastases in the first capillary net that traps them after they detach from their parent growth, but instead migrate until they reach a particular organ and only then give rise to metastases.[2,3]

Clearly, the processes of detachment from the tumor mass, survival in blood, lodging in the proper capillary net of the proper organ and growth in the organ are not matters of chance. Instead they seem to be the result of innate properties of certain cancer cells and certain cancer cells only. If, in fact, cancers arise from single cells, it is reasonable to expect all their daughters to share a common genotype and to exhibit common properties. Since the ability to metastasize is a property exhibited by certain cells in a cancer only, an explanation must be sought as to why that subpopulation of cancer cells differs from the rest. There are various possibilities. These cells may have undergone mutation, one which differentiates them from the rest of a malignant mass by permitting them to metastasize.

A second possibility might be that these cells have *differentiated* from the parent cancer cell population. Differentiation, in the biological or developmental sense, means that certain aspects of the genotype of cells are either suppressed or permitted to be expressed. All normal cells of the body share a common genotype. Yet, clearly, all are not alike. Nerve differs from muscle, gut, skin and so forth, in ways so striking and convincing that no illustration is needed to help explain the differences. In each of these cell types portions of the common genotype are suppressed, permitting expression only of the rest. Conceivably, a portion of cancer cells' genotype, normally suppressed, is derepressed, and the result is a cell which may migrate and begin a new growth.

A third possibility might be that all cancer cells possess the capacity to metastasize, but that only a few express this because their microenvironment permits it. This explanation supposes that the microenvironment within or around cancers differs significantly and, indeed, this may be so. Certainly oxygenation and concentration of nutritional materials can differ within regions of cancers, exposure to host antibodies can be greater near vessels than far from them and products released from dead or dying cancer cells may be more concentrated in various tumor regions than others.

No evidence distinguishing absolutely among these and possibly other alternatives exists, but it is important that the issue eventually be decided. Local and regional disease can, even now in many instances, be controlled or "cured" by available non-surgical means as well as by surgery. Cancer deaths most often are due to disseminated disease, which itself is due to metastasis. However, the *means* of best controlling the metastatic process will in all probability be determined by understanding the mechanisms underlying the process. If metastasis is the result of a specific genotype, the process will be controlled best by killing metastasizing cells or those with metastatic potential. If, alternatively, metastasis is the consequence of differentiation, means may be developed which artificially might suppress the genes responsible for it. But, if it is due to a permissive effect of cancer microenvironment, then alteration in tumor environment may be effective in controlling it.

Whatever the explanation of changes in tumor cells as tumors grow, these changes substantially influence clinical practice.

Clinical Implications. The size a tumor attains prior to therapy influences greatly the manner in which it must be treated and the results that are likely to be obtained. Larger tumors require more aggressive therapy and frequently, even then, do not yield to treatment. However, the converse of this idea probably is the more important principle in current thinking; that is, the smaller the tumor, the lower the dose necessary to control it at any level of statistical probability. In terms of radiotherapy, damage to adjacent normal tissues limits the amount of treatment that can be administered. Irradiation therefore is more effective against a smaller tumor because less normal tissue damage must be inflicted in order to be likely to cure it. In terms of chemotherapy, where currently available drugs are limited to their narrow differential effect on normal and cancerous tissue, success will more frequently occur when tumor burden is small.

Definitive Radiotherapy. Considerable evidence exists to support the concept that the dose required to control a tumor is a function of the size of that tumor.[1] Less dose is required to control disease microscopic in size, than to control disease that is clinically evident. And within the group of tumors that can be measured grossly, larger tumors require higher doses than do smaller tumors. Translated into other terms, microscopic amounts of breast cancer which are adjacent to critical normal tissues such as spinal cord can be eradicated by radiotherapy while taking less than a 5% risk of damaging spinal cord. In contrast, a 5-cm tumor requires doses entailing greater than a 50% risk of inducing myelopathy. Precisely how important physical size *per se* is in relation to associated factors discussed elsewhere in this book is unclear; however, since tumor size is a relatively simple parameter to assess, it is frequently used as a guide although it may be only an index of some other factors.

Adjuvant Radiotherapy. Whatever the cause, it is quite clear that radiotherapy is most effective when used against small tumor burdens. For example, as a postsurgical procedure, it deals with minute amounts of tumor the surgeon cannot detect grossly, but which, from experience, are likely to have been left behind. Several sites in the body lend themselves to such treatment.

As described in Chapter 2, anaplastic primary brain tumors tend to extend greatly throughout cerebral matter, thereby effectively precluding total surgical removal. However, by excising as much tumor as is commensurate with retaining neurologic function, the remaining burden is more likely to be controlled by subsequent radiation therapy than would have been the case if the entire tumor were there. Similarly, postoperative irradiation frequently is recommended for more advanced, more aggressive tumors arising in head and neck sites and the colorectum.

Alternatively, radiotherapy can be given preoperatively. In such cases, the same radiobiologic principles apply; however, the clinical effect differs. In essence, surgery still removes the bulk of the tumor and radiation sterilizes the peripheral fronds. The sequencing of radiotherapy before surgery, however, allows this method to be used when tumor is adherent to non-resectable structures. Doses similar to those used postoperatively are employed, and while they usually do not sterilize the entire tumor mass, they do produce sufficient shrinkage to permit total resection. Irradiation may convert an inoperable situation into an operable one. An additional benefit of preoperative irradiation, at least in theory, is that irradiated tumor cells liberated into the bloodstream during surgery are less likely to be able to implant elsewhere and form a metastasis. Planned, combined irradiation and surgery is a standard method of treatment for some advanced tumors of the head and neck, cervix, endometrium, and urinary bladder, and soft tissue sarcomas.

Chemotherapy. Size of the tumor burden substantially affects the ability of chemotherapy to produce a desired result too. Cancer for cancer, eradication of disease is more likely when less tumor is present.

The Experimental Evidence. The mechanism of chemotherapy-induced response was demonstrated clearly by Skipper et al.[5,6] in a murine model. Using a transplantable tumor, they noted that the time between tumor transplantation and death of host depended upon the number of tumor cells transplanted. The larger the number transplanted, the shorter was the time between transplant and death. They could show, further, that treatment of tumor before transplantation with given doses of antineoplastic drug, extended length of life between transplant and death. In other words, even though the same number of drug treated and untreated cells were transplanted to identical host mice, animals receiving drug-treated cells lived longer. Since there were no changes in tumor cell generation time, this suggests that only a proportion of drug-treated cells were effective in producing tumor. It therefore follows that *proliferative capacity* in some treated cells was destroyed by the drug. The action of these drugs appears quite similar to that of radiation; namely, cell sterilization of a *proportion* of a cell population. If radiation and antineoplastic drug doses sterilize only a proportion of any cell population (however large), some cells with reproductive potential will always be left after treatment. Tumor *control* occurs when cell kill reduces the cell number to a level that can be handled by the host's own defenses. Precisely what this level is remains unknown; however, it must be below that at which tumor clinically is detectable. Indeed, while most patients who experience a complete remission (i.e. all their measurable disease vanishes) subsequently relapse, some patients have remained disease-free for prolonged periods and appear cured. On the other hand, for many types of tumors, partial remissions where disease clinically is still evident do not appear to be of value.

Clinical Applications. As discussed previously, the unique value of chemotherapy is its ability to act effectively *throughout* the body. Such actions against metastatic disease have earned chemotherapy a place as one of the three main forms of anticancer treatment. And yet, when drugs are used against cancers, the amount of disease is predetermined and usually large. However, there are situations wherein chemotherapy can be administered when disease burden is relatively low.

After surgery for advanced ovarian carcinoma, residual tumor frequently is present. Depending upon initial extent of disease, either macroscopic or microscopic amounts of cancer may remain, but in either case, subsequent chemotherapy will have to deal with less disease than was present prior to surgery. Many experts therefore advise removing as much disease as possible, even when the lesion is not totally resectable, before administering chemotherapy.

Elective Chemotherapy. Since chemotherapy is less likely to be effective against grossly evident tumors than microscopic size, subclinical disease, thought recently has turned to elective administration of chemotherapy for suspected, but unproven metastases.

Several conditions must be met for elective chemotherapy to be successful. *First*, the disease being treated must be prone to producing occult spread which is not encompassed by conventional primary treatment. Lung tumors provide a good example. *Second*, a drug (or drugs) must be available which has (have) *substantial* cytotoxic effect against the tumor. Oat cell carcinomas of lung qualify in this respect, but the remaining majority of lung tumors, squamous cell carcinomas, adenocarcinomas and large cell undifferentiated carcinomas do not. Effectiveness, undoubtedly, is the crux of the problem, but also the aspect most difficult to assess. When patients are treated for metastatic disease, positive influence of the drug is measured by regression in the size of disease. When treatment is given for *presumed* metastatic disease, the concept of clinical regression cannot apply. A positive influence of the drug can only be measured by decreased recurrence rates or increased survival, relative to a population that does not receive the drug. An association between ability to effect regression and ability to decrease recurrence rates (or increase survival) is often presumed but may not, in fact, be real. Still more complex is the question of clinical regression versus sterilization of disease. Hormones produce the former without causing the latter. If adjuvant therapy merely causes regression without effecting sterilization of disease, the same number of patients will eventually suffer a recurrence when disease escapes control, and at least some patients will have to endure side effects needlessly. Thus, for elective adjuvant treatment to be truly valuable, it must actually eradicate disease. *Third*, elective adjuvant therapy must not interfere with primary treatment. Were adjuvant therapy 100% effective against subclinical disease, it would nevertheless be contraindicated, if it prevented effective therapy of the primary measurable cancer. Precise combinations of basic and adjuvant therapy that yield optimum results for different types of tumor are the subject of many current investigations.

The State of the Art. Adjuvant chemotherapy has been proven to be effective in some situations, and there are suggestions that it may be effective in others. As previously noted, elective chemotherapy appears to be changing the prognosis for some women who have breast cancer, particularly when they are at high risk of recurrence because of the aggressive nature of their disease.

Much of the evidence for the efficacy of adjuvant chemotherapy has been gained from experience with tumors that occur in the pediatric age group. Depending upon type and stage of disease, the appropriate regimen varies, but it is quite clear that administering adjuvant therapy is considered "standard management" of certain diseases.[7] For example, Wilms' tumor (a cancer composed of primitive renal parenchymal cells) initially is treated by radical nephrectomy. If tumor penetrates the renal capsule, irradiation of all invaded areas is added to secure local control. All patients are then placed on elective combination chemotherapy (actinomycin D and vincristine). With such management, more than 90% of patients who do not have detectable distant metastases at the time their disease is diagnosed, are cured.

Combined Radiotherapy and Chemotherapy. Effective use of radiotherapy and chemotherapy as adjuvants is not limited to situations wherein surgery is the prime mode of management. Either modality can be used as an adjuvant to the other. There is evidence that oat cell carcinomas are being controlled more effectively by administering chemotherapy for unproven, but presumed, distant metastases, while using radiation therapy to treat grossly evident disease. Elective chemotherapy in the treatment of Ewing's sarcoma of bone is directed against distant metastases, while radiotherapy is used to locally control primary disease. Somewhat of a reversal in roles sometimes occurs when advanced Hodgkin's disease is treated by a combination of chemotherapy and radiotherapy. In one form of such management, multidrug chemotherapy is initially administered. Then as a planned second phase, even though the patient's disease is hoped to have gone into clinical remission, relatively low levels of radiation are administered to sites which initially contained gross disease on the presumption that non-detectable amounts persist, since recurrences following chemotherapy alone frequently are in sites that contained macroscopic disease before treatment.

Furthermore, radiotherapy and chemotherapy can be used in conjunction as adjuvants to surgery. For many years, radical surgery (often amputation) was considered essential to control sarcomas. However, it is now known that irradiation of a wide margin around more moderate surgical procedures produces equivalent local control with far better function and cosmesis. Moreover, the addition of elective chemotherapy appears to decrease likelihood of failure due to distant metastases.

References

1. Fidler, I.J.: In *Cancer: A Comprehensive Treatise*. Vol. 4. Frederick F. Becker (Ed.). New York, Plenum Press, 1975.
2. Nicolson, G.L.: Experimental Tumor Metastases: Characteristics and Organ Specificity. Bioscience 28:441–447, 1978.
3. Nicolson, G.L., and Brunson, K.W.: Specificity of Arrest, Survival, and Growth of Selected Metastatic Variant Cell Lines. Cancer Res. 38:4105–4111, 1978.
4. Research Plan for Radiation Oncology: Tumor Dose-Time-Volume, Committee for Radiation Oncol. Studies. Cancer 37:2056–2061, 1976.
5. Skipper, H.E., Schabel, F.M. Jr., and Wilcox, W.S.: Experimental Evaluation of Anticancer Agents XIII. Ca. Chemother. Rep. 35:1–111, 1964.
6. Skipper, H.E., Schabel, F.M. Jr., and Wilcox, W.S.: XIV. Further Study of Certain Basic Concepts Underlying Chemotherapy of Leukemia. Ca. Chemother. Rep. 45:5–28, 1965.
7. Exelby, P.E.: Solid Tumors in Children: Wilms' Tumor, Neuroblastoma and Soft Tissue Sarcomas. Ca—A Cancer J. for Clinicians 28:146–163, 1978.

11

EFFECT OF BLOOD SUPPLY

Because cancers grow faster than their blood supply, tumor cells must compete for their needs. Those cells most distant from capillaries get little oxygen and probably little nutrient, too. Moreover, evidence exists to demonstrate that blood which does flow through tumors, flows sluggishly; tumor capillaries often follow a tortuous course, and their many twists and turns retard flow. Thus, circulation within tumors is inadequate and this inadequacy profoundly affects tumor growth.

Deficiencies of circulation may, in a sense, benefit the untreated host. Severely oxygen-deficient tumor cells are unable to reproduce and proliferate. In the untreated host, they cannot be part of the *growing* cancer and so do not threaten the life of the host. In fact, death as a result of severe hypoxia or anoxia is likely to be a principal means by which cells are lost from cancers.

Inadequate circulation also modifies the outcome of therapy. Response to treatment is controlled to an important degree by the tumor's blood supply. Oxygen deficiency poses a major obstacle to successful radiation therapy and the factors which lead to nutrient deficiency act as an obstacle to chemotherapy. However, sluggish circulation through the capillaries of a tumor may be of benefit in treating cancers with hyperthermia or with hyperthermia and radiation together.

This chapter deals with the problems posed by inadequate circulation, the effect they have on various therapies, and the means being tried and sought to solve them.

Oxygen-Deficient Tumor Regions. The distance from blood vessel to tumor cell influences that cell's metabolism. If cells are too far away, they become hypoxic and those most distant, for practical purposes,

157

are anoxic. Warburg[1] has calculated that cells more than 150 microns from capillaries carrying blood at normal oxygen tension, will be anoxic, and Thomlinson and Gray[2] have shown on histologic preparations, that cells more than 200 microns distant from feeding capillaries are necrotic. These necrotic cells coalesce and form necrotic regions such as are seen in many kinds of tumors particularly carcinomas (Chap. 9). Although large tumors are commonly pictured as having relatively large necrotic regions, small tumors may have small regions composed of severely hypoxic, even anoxic cells. These small foci can influence the results of therapy and their influence can be quite disproportionate to their size.

The Effect of Oxygen Deprived Cells on Radiotherapy. Briefly stated, oxygen deprivation confers *resistance* to most common forms of radiation therapy, x rays, gamma rays and electrons. Hypoxic and/or anoxic tumor cells are not usually killed by doses of these radiations that are lethal to well-aerated tumor cells and, more important, to *normal* cells of the tissue in which the cancer happens to be situated. Normal tissues, in contrast to cancers, generally are well-aerated and contain no hypoxic or anoxic regions. The degree of resistance conferred by oxygen deprivation varies according to specific circumstances. As a general rule, however, hypoxic cells are between 2.5 and 3.0 times *less* sensitive to x rays, gamma rays or electrons than are well-aerated cells. To destroy foci of hypoxic cancer cells doses between 2 and 3 times the tolerance of normal tissue have to be used. Such doses bring about unacceptable levels of complications and cannot be used in clinical practice.

Clinical Variation. Although inadequacies of blood supply affect all tumors, in certain circumstances the problem is more or less pronounced. To some extent, the pattern of tumor growth denotes the adequacy of cellular blood supply. Whether tumors which generate an abundant blood supply are permitted to grow outward from their surface of origin, in an exophytic manner, or if exophytic tumors have a propensity to *elicit* neovascularization is unknown, but the association of exophytic tumors and adequate blood supply certainly exists. In contrast, burrowing ulcerative tumors characteristically incorporate a relatively poorer blood supply. These factors profoundly influence management as will be discussed shortly.

It is important to understand that one must measure blood supply delivered to tumor cells, not the degree of vasculature which encompasses or passes through tumor. In this regard some common jargon is misleading. For example, when an angiogram demonstrates substantial contrast enhancement of a lesion, a so-called tumor blush, the accepted interpretation is that the tumor has an abundant vascular supply. However, one cannot conclude that individual cells of that tumor are well-oxygenated. Transport to individual cells requires an efficient *microvasculature*; vessels that can be seen on an angiogram are of macroscopic size and their presence does not necessarily indicate that an adequate microvasculature is also present.

In addition to a well-developed system of transport (the microvasculature) tumors require an adequate carrier of oxygen and nutrients within the system and blood itself fulfills this role. Consequently, independent of the adequacy of the vasculature, when insufficient numbers of red blood cells are circulating, the tumor cannot be well oxygenated. Uncorrected anemia therefore decreases likelihood of successful therapy. Bush et al.[3] demonstrated that women who received irradiation for advanced cervical carcinoma fared significantly worse if their hemoglobin levels were below 12 mg% than those with higher levels. Furthermore, in a prospective study, correction of anemia in another group of patients resulted in less frequent pelvic failure and increased cure rates. However, the precise degree of anemia which is significant and the extent to which transfusion can compensate for this problem remains to be elucidated.

Fractionated Irradiation. Because oxygen deficiency, to a greater or lesser degree, is an unavoidable fact in oncology, means have been sought to circumvent or overcome it. The method most commonly used at present, attacks oxygen deficient foci of tumor indirectly, by fractionating radiotherapy. The total dose is split up and delivered at intervals over a period of several days to several weeks. Daily doses of 200 rads often are used although considerable variation is possible, depending upon the extent of tumor and intent of treatment. When cancers are irradiated in this fashion, the first few fractions probably kill only well-aerated cells, normal and neoplastic. Oxygen deprived cells which exist only in the cancer, are too resistant to be destroyed. Nevertheless, this *does* reduce the total number of living cells in the cancer so that after a few fractions, fewer cells compete for oxygen diffusing from tumor capillaries. Cells which were hypoxic because demand for oxygen exceeded supply, can improve in aeration because supply becomes more nearly equal to demand. Concurrently, the overall degree of cellular resistance to radiation diminishes, because resistance is a result of hypoxia and not an intrinsic, immutable quality of hypoxic cells. Experimental evidence exists to demonstrate this concept.

Reoxygenation. Van Putten and Kallman[1] determined the proportion of hypoxic cells in a transplantable mouse sarcoma of spontaneous origin at a specific size and age. In their system, under their conditions, 14% of the cells were hypoxic. They determined the proportion of hypoxic cells in this tumor after various *fractionated* radiotherapy regimens. One group of tumors was exposed to daily fractions of irradiation, Monday through Friday for a total of five fractions. The hypoxic proportion was determined on the following Monday and was 18%. Another group of tumors was given four fractions, Monday through Thursday, and the hypoxic proportion, determined the next day, Friday, was 14%.

After both these regimens the hypoxic proportion was nearly that of an untreated tumor, namely 14%. The radiation doses that were used kill well-aerated tumor cells, but probably do not kill hypoxic ones. If all hypoxic cells had remained hypoxic and resistant while well-aerated ones were killed, the *proportion* of hypoxic cells can only have increased. Since this did not happen, some hypoxic cells must have become radiosensitive. The explanation most commonly accepted is

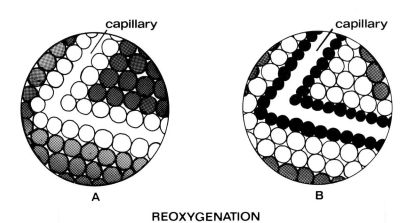

REOXYGENATION

Fig. 11–1.   *Schematic representation of reoxygenation following irradiation. A. Unshaded cells are near capillary, well oxygenated and relatively radiosensitive. Shaded cells, distant from the capillary, are hypoxic and relatively radioresistant. B. Radiation has killed darkly colored cells near capillary allowing oxygen to diffuse further from capillary, thereby reoxygenating some previously hypoxic cells.*

that during these radiation regimens, some hypoxic cells *reoxygenated*, i.e., reverted to oxygenated cells (Fig. 11–1).

In theory, at least, if the course of radiation therapy is sufficiently prolonged, all hypoxic cells can become aerated, and the probability of killing them would then be as good as killing cancer cells which were well-aerated all along. There are, however, difficulties which interfere with successful clinical application of this concept. At present, there is no *conclusive* proof that hypoxic human cancer cells reoxygenate, or if they do, how quickly this occurs. This in turn precludes precise determination of *how prolonged* a course of radiation therapy needs to be, for surely that depends on how swiftly reoxygenation occurs and how complete it is in a given period of time.

Nevertheless, several considerations strongly suggest that reoxygenation of *human* cancers must occur. Calculations indicate that even if only a small fraction of cancer cells normally are hypoxic (less than 1%) and spared from lethal radiation injury because of it, virtually *all* treated cancers would locally recur in the remaining lifetime of affected persons. Yet, recurrence within an irradiated field is uncommon. This indicates that either hypoxic cells are not present in most human cancers (quite unlikely) or that, in most instances, reoxygenation takes place.

Hypoxia and Recovery. In general, oxygen deficiency protects hypoxic cancer cells because it confers resistance to radiation damage. However, oxygen deficiency has another effect which is detrimental to irradiated hypoxic cells.

When irradiated, all cells, well-aerated or hypoxic, may be damaged. Hypoxic cells, although resistant, are not spared entirely, even though *less* damage is done to them than is done to well-aerated cells by given radiation doses. Sublethal damage is potentially reparable and cells may, under proper conditions, fully recover from it. If cells recover, they tolerate subsequent radiation damage as well as unirradiated cells of the same kind. If cells do not recover, their ability to withstand subsequent irradiation is decreased. Essential requirements for recovery include time (it is not instantaneous) and *oxygen*. During a course of fractionated radiotherapy, well-aerated cells are damaged, but, between fractions of radiation, recover. Hypoxic cells are more difficult to damage owing to their hypoxia-produced lack of sensitivity, but they cannot recover from that damage. As treatment progresses, surviving well-aerated cells constantly purge themselves of sublethal damage. But surviving hypoxic cells merely accumulate damage; in time, lethal levels may be reached. This, in fact, is likely to be one of the chief reasons for the success of *fractionated* radiation therapy. It *spares* normal tissues which are well-aerated and can undergo repair at the expense of hypoxic cells which cannot.

Clearly, the presence of hypoxic cells greatly complicates the radiation oncologist's task. Prolonged fractionation can—at least in theory—make these cells vulnerable to irradiation, but the process which makes them vulnerable, may also make them dangerous. Cells which (1) readily reoxygenate, become sensitive and are sterilized, (2) do not reoxygenate, cannot recover and die of accumulated damage or (3) do not reoxygenate and die of chronic anoxia are all effectively controlled after a course of fractionated irradiation. However, hypoxic cancer cells which reoxygenate at or near the completion of treatment may not receive sufficient radiation to be sterilized. In a sense, fractionated radiotherapy rescues them from chronic hypoxia caused death. Because they have reoxygenated, they may begin again to grow and eventually manifest themselves as a recurrent tumor. Consequently, direct methods which effectively destroy hypoxic cells have been sought.

Three separate approaches exist to deal with oxygen deficient cells. The first attempts to add oxygen to hypoxic foci. The second attempts to minimize the problem by developing oxygen-independent radiation techniques. The third attempts to develop chemical substitutes for oxygen.

Hyperbaric Oxygen. Because oxygen deficiency has been ascribed to an inadequate supply of oxygen, early approaches attempted to increase capillary oxygen. One which elicited substantial clinical interest was termed "hyperbaric oxygenation."[5] In short, the amount of oxygen in blood (the oxygen tension) is controlled by the amount of oxygen inspired. "Normal" oxygenation results when air at atmospheric pressure is breathed. Increased oxygenation is expected if the amount of inspired oxygen is increased (air is 21% oxygen; this can be increased to 100% oxygen) and/or if the pressure of the inspired oxygen is increased. During clinical trials both were done. Patients breathed pure oxygen, usually at 3 atmospheres of pressure, before and during irradiation, a technique that should increase the oxygen concentration in blood about 20 times. Clearly, if this happened, there would be more oxygen in capillaries and more available for all cells.

The results of clinical trials fell into two categories. Some showed striking success. There were many fewer recurrences in the irradiated field in patients breathing oxygen at high pressure than in those breathing air. Others found little (if any) difference. For years this discrepancy went unexplained and the method itself, open to question, was not vigorously pursued. Recently, however, a difference between the trials has emerged which may account for the observed difference. Good results often occurred when patients were not anesthetized during treatment, while the method often failed when patients were anesthetized using sodium pentobarbital. It turns out that the anesthetic is a powerful radiation protector and may have protected the cancers in some of the trials. Consequently, hyperbaric therapy is being re-examined and may yet be quite useful.

Heavy Particle Irradiation. Heavy, highly charged particles provide a physical solution to the problem of hypoxia. As a general rule, when these densely ionizing radiations are used, there is little difference in response of oxygen-deficient and well-aerated cells. Neutrons, although uncharged, interact in tissue to produce protons, relatively massive, charged particles and, therefore, indirectly yield similar results. Some clinical centers now use neutrons in place of X or gamma radiations to diminish the oxygen effect. Catterall et al.[6] reported a prospective randomized trial of neutron irradiation, compared with X or gamma irradiation, in patients having advanced head and neck tumors. Both in terms of frequency of complete regression and of frequency of *persistent* local control, the neutron group fared significantly better. In other patients[7] having two similar metastatic lesions, one treated with neutrons and the other treated by X or gamma rays, control of the former *always* exceeded that of the latter. In no case did the neutron treated lesion show less regression than its counterpart. While oxygen-deficient cells irradiated by neutrons (or more properly, the protons they release in tissue) are less radioresistant than similar cells irradiated by X or gamma rays, a small but significant oxygen-effect remains. The use of atomic nuclei (atoms stripped of their electrons) at least in theory, can reduce the oxygen-effect to negligible proportions; when irradiated with sufficiently heavy, charged particles, well aerated and oxygen deficient cells should respond in the same way.

Clinical trials now in progress using negative pi meson (negative pion) beams are an ingenious variation of this theme. While these radiations are neither massive nor highly charged, they are "captured" by atoms in tissues and these atoms subsequently explode. Their disintegrating nuclei shower massive, highly charged fragments into the surrounding tissue and act as massive charged radiations. Not enough data have yet been gathered to decide how effective the method will be.

Radiosensitizing Drugs. Radiosensitizing drugs provide a pharmacologic solution to hypoxia. These chemicals enhance damage done by ionizing radiation and fall into two categories, "true" and "false" sensitizers. Cytotoxic action of true sensitizers and radiation are *synergistic,* while those of false sensitizers and radiation are merely *additive.* Unless the sensitizer can selectively increase damage to tumor cells, it is of no more value than an increased dose of irradiation and is more difficult to administer.

Several types of radiosensitizers exist and their relative efficacy and potential varies. The chemotherapeutic agents actinomycin-D, adriamycin, methotrexate and 5-fluorouracil, at least in vitro, potentiate the effect of radiotherapy. Whether true radiosensitization occurs is unclear; the effect may result simply from the addition of the respective actions of the drug and radiotherapy. Furthermore, the clinical value of these drugs as sensitizers is limited by the concurrent action on normal tissue.

Halogenated pyrimidines such as 5-bromodeoxyuridine (BUdR) also act as sensitizers. Structurally similar to thymidine, these compounds are incorporated into the DNA chain *during* cell replication, and in some as yet unexplained manner, impair the integrity of the chain. Cells with this aberrant DNA suffer greater x ray damage than other cells. Tumor cells having a high mitotic rate can acquire appreciable amounts of this fragile DNA before the less active surrounding normal cells are affected. Unfortunately, dehalogenation of the drug by the liver necessitates direct intra-arterial administration. Despite this limitation, patients have been treated in this fashion,[8] although to date no significant clinical benefit has been shown.

The most promising type of radiosensitizer is represented by the electron affinic compounds such as metronidazole (Flagyl) and misonidazole (Ro–07–0582; Roche). These drugs substitute for oxygen in the free-radical reactions which promote radiation-induced damage and thereby minimize the effect of hypoxia. Clearly they are effective in experimental models.[9]

As might be expected, the pharmacology of these compounds has received close scrutiny in an attempt to understand them better and improve their radiosensitizing properties. Structurally, they are quite similar. Metronidazole is a nitroimidazole having its nitro group at the "5" carbon position, while misonidazole is a 2-nitroimidazole. Both drugs can be given orally, are widely distributed throughout the body, and have the relatively long biologic half-lives[9] required to permit diffusion of drug to the tumor. Unfortunately, these compounds are not innocuous and neurotoxicity, manifested primarily by sensory peripheral neuropathy, limits the amount and frequency with which they can be given.

Urtasun[10] reported a prospective randomized trial of the value of metronidazole plus irradiation in patients who had glioblastoma multiforme. Although this study can be criticized for the low dose of irradiation that was given, there was a statistically significant improvement in survival for those patients who received the drug.

Misonidazole has even greater potential. On theoretical grounds and in experimental systems, it is more effective than metronidazole. Nationwide trials of misonidazole are now under way to test its clinical value.

Other types of anticancer therapy are also affected by tumor circulation, although comparatively little information on the subject exists. While the effect of hypoxia is generally not considered in chemotherapeutic management, the difficulty of getting appreciable amounts of drug to the tumor generally is appreciated.

The Effect of Blood Supply on Chemotherapy. The limitations of blood circulation within tumors adversely affects chemotherapeutic management. Drugs with antineoplastic properties, tend to be composed of large molecules and difficulties in transport to and diffusion within tumors, previously described for oxygen, apply at least equally well to these drugs. Some tumors are sufficiently chemosensitive to exhibit marked regression from the relatively small amounts of drug that can be delivered by the disorganized tumor vasculature; however, the most impressive responses to chemotherapy, if not cures, are seen most frequently with the non-solid hematologic neoplasms (leukemias, lymphomas), where the disease is immersed in the vascular or lymphatic streams, and in choriocarcinomas of women, which are derived from tissue that specializes in producing abundant vascular channels.

For a given type of tumor the probability of successful treatment is inversely proportional to its size and therefore its reliance upon a disordered, inadequate vasculature. Even diseases that are frequently sensitive to chemotherapy, such as lymphomas, tend to relapse at sites that initially contained bulky disease. However, the amounts of drug which are administered cannot be increased blindly in an attempt to overwhelm these circulatory barriers.

Unfortunately, drugs administered systemically by either oral, intramuscular or intravenous routes are delivered at least equally well to many normal tissues. The likelihood of successful therapy, wherein the tumor is destroyed but no complications of treatment are produced, depends on the tumor being more sensitive to the drug than is any other exposed tissue. The problem is compounded by the existence of so called "sanctuary sites" (e.g. brain) into which most chemotherapeutic agents cannot penetrate. Even highly sensitive neoplasms such as acute lymphocytic leukemia are protected from chemotherapeutic action in these sites.

Chemotherapeutic solutions to the problem of limited circulation basically seek to increase the amount of drug delivered to the tumor without increasing the amount of drug delivered to normal tissues. Direct infusion of drug into tumor, delivers the entire administered amount to the tumor, while normal tissues are exposed to a fractional amount because of dilution by the blood stream. In clinical practice, however, this technique seldom is used since it requires invasive techniques of drug administration (with their attendant risk) and because tumors frequently have more than one source of vascular supply (which immediately dilutes the drug).

The unique anatomy of the extremities permits tumors of the arm and leg to be treated by perfusion therapy. In essence, this technique isolates the affected region from the systemic circulation by means of tourniquets placed in the axillary or femoral regions. Because most chemosensitive normal tissues remain untreated, doses several times larger than can be given on a systemic basis are well tolerated. This method is limited by the relative rarity of tumors in the extremities, the unavoidable seepage of some drug beyond the tourniquet and the unavoidable release of some drug from the affected limb to the systemic circulation once the tourniquet is removed.

Tumors, which cannot be isolated anatomically, can sometimes be isolated pharmacologically. The prime example of such systems is the sequential use of methotrexate and folinic acid. The antimetabolite methotrexate acts to block formation of tetrahydrofolic acid, a necessary precursor of the essential dietary factor folic acid. In practice, inhibition caused by methotrexate is so effective that once the drug becomes bound to the cell, the reaction is nearly irreversible. On the other hand, folinic acid can replace the unproduced tetrahydrofolic acid and thereby prevent cell death. Clinically, massive doses of methotrexate are used to overcome deficiencies in tumor circulation and bind to both normal and abnormal cells. Folinic acid (citrovorum factor) is subsequently administered, but only normal cells are rescued. Although the mechanism of selective rescue is unproven, a likely explanation is the preferential delivery of folinic acid to normal tissues, which have adequate circulation, as compared to tumor tissue, which does not. This method, however, is limited to those neoplasms which are sensitive to methotrexate.

The Effect of Circulation on Hyperthermia. The inadequacy of circulation within tumors does not always interfere with therapy; treatment of cancer by heat is aided by limitations of vasculature. Although hyperthermia is not frequently considered a prime method of anticancer therapy, it can kill tumors. Recently, a firm biologic appreciation of the effect of heat on neoplasms has been gained.[11,12] Hypoxic cells suffer greater damage from heat than do well-oxygenated cells. Thus, hypoxic foci created by insufficient blood supply pose no difficulty in hyperthermic therapy. Furthermore, the disorganized vasculature proves intrinsically detrimental to the neoplasm. LeVeen et al.[13] have demonstrated the inability of these vessels to dissipate heat. Through various means, temperature gradients of 5° to 9°C between tumor and normal tissues can be generated and tumor regression or necrosis produced.

Adjuvant Surgery. Although the rationale for surgical management of tumors exceeds the scope of this book, it should be noted that deficiencies of tumor blood supply do not diminish the effectiveness of surgical therapy. Unlike radiotherapy or chemotherapy which are most effective against small, even microscopic tumors, surgical therapy is most effective against well-demarcated masses. Thus, various combinations, such as radiotherapeutic sterilization of the periphery of a tumor combined with surgical extirpation of the central core are becoming increasingly common in clinical practice. Head and neck cancer and "barrel shaped" carcinoma of the cervix are examples of lesions that benefit from such treatment.

References

1. Warburg, O.: The Metabolism of Tumors. London, Constable, 1930, p. 6.
2. Thomlinson, R.H., and Gray, L.H.: Histological Structure of Some Human Lung Cancers and the Possible Implications for Radiotherapy. Br. J. Cancer 9:539–549, 1955.

3. Bush, R.S., et al.: Definitive Evidence for Hypoxic Cells Influencing Cure in Cancer Therapy. Br. J. Cancer 37:302–306, 1978.
4. Van Putten, L.M., and Kallman, R.F.: Oxygenation Status of a Transplantable Tumor During Fractionated Radiotherapy. J. Nat'l. Ca. Inst. 40:441–451, 1968.
5. Vaeth, J.M. (Ed.): Hyperbaric Oxygen and Radiation Therapy of Cancer. Berkeley, CA, McCutchan Publishing Corporation, 1966.
6. Catterall, M., Sutherland, I., and Bewley, D.K.: First Results of Randomized Clinical Trial of Fast Neutrons Compared with X or Gamma Rays in Treatment of Advanced Tumors of the Head and Neck. Br. Med. J. 2:653–656, 1975.
7. Catterall, M.: Radiology Now, Fast Neutrons—Clinical Requirements. Br. J. Radiol. 49:203–205, 1976.
8. Bagshaw, M.A., et al.: Intra-Arterial 5-Bromodeoxyuridine and X-ray Therapy. Am. J. Roentgenol. 99:886–894, 1967.
9. Committee for Radiation Oncology Studies: Radiation Sensitizers. Cancer 37:2062–2071, 1976.
10. Urtasun, R., et al.: Radiation and High Dose Metronidazole (Flagyl) in Supratentorial Glioblastomas. N. Engl. J. Med. 294:1364–1367, 1976.
11. Committee for Radiation Oncology Studies: Hyperthermia in the Treatment of The Cancer Patient. Cancer 37:2075–2083, 1976.
12. Proceedings of the International Symposium on Cancer Therapy by Hyperthermia and Radiation, Washington, D.C., April 28–30, 1975, American College of Radiology.
13. LeVeen, H.H., et al.: Tumor Eradication by Radiofrequency Therapy. J.A.M.A. 235:2196–2200, 1976.

12
EFFECT OF SITE OF DISEASE

The site at which a tumor arises and the sites to which it spreads are key factors in oncology. *First*, the site of origin influences both histologic cell type (Chap. 5) and degree of differentiation (Chap. 6). *Second*, the anatomic site may promote specific growth patterns, such as central vs. peripheral tumors or exophytic vs. ulcerative tumors. In turn, these patterns often determine both typical symptoms associated with tumors at that site and likelihood of lymphatic or hematogenous dissemination. *Third*, the areas involved by tumor often decide the basic principles of treatment and may restrict its expectations. *Fourth*, involvement of specific anatomic sites may limit acceptable methods of therapy and may demand that treatment be administered on an emergency basis. *Last*, prognosis depends largely upon sites of involvement. For these reasons, the effect of the site of disease is elaborated in this chapter.

Patterns of Disease. Tumors of nearly every organ exhibit characteristic spatial patterns. Whether tumors arise centrally, peripherally, laterally, medially, proximally or distally occurs not by chance. For example, tumors of the anterior tongue tend to grow along the *lateral* margins, carcinomas of the prostate begin in the *posterior* lobe, colorectal carcinomas tend to be *distal*. In organs which give rise to more than one histologic type of tumor, there can be different patterns of distribution for each type. Squamous cell carcinomas of the esophagus are *proximal*, while adenocarcinomas are *distal*. Similarly, squamous cell carcinomas of the lung are *central*, close to the mediastinum, while adenocarcinomas are more likely to be *peripheral*.

Site also can affect the manner in which tumor grows. Carcinomas of

169

the pharyngeal tonsil frequently are exophytic, while carcinomas of the floor of the mouth tend to be infiltrative in nature. Because of differences in blood supply to these different patterns of tumor growth (Chap. 11), they can present substantially different problems in management.

Effect of Distribution Within a Given Site. The specific site of disease also determines the symptoms which accompany it and the likelihood of its detection. If the site is easily accessible or has a function in which minute changes easily can be detected, the lesion frequently can be detected early. For example, cytologic analysis of scrapings from the uterine cervix permits early detection of tumors arising in that organ. At present, approximately two-thirds of cervical carcinomas are discovered before they have had a chance to become invasive. Similarly, a carcinoma of the vocal cord gives rise to hoarseness so rapidly that it frequently is detected in an early stage. On the other hand, ovarian carcinomas grow in a non-accessible region, rarely are detectable by changes in ovarian function and, as a result, usually are advanced when diagnosed.

For larger organs, the precise location of a lesion within an organ can be important. A tumor originating in the body of the pancreas can attain large size before giving rise to symptoms. However, a similar lesion arising in the head of the pancreas, rapidly may occlude the draining duct, give rise to symptoms and thereby be detected relatively early.

In some large organs, symptoms differ when the tumor occupies different regions. A colon carcinoma characteristically produces obstruction and change in bowel habits when it is in the descending left colon, but usually manifests itself by signs of associated blood loss when it is in the ascending right side.

Moreover, these differences in position can have profound impact on treatment. A brain tumor in a clinically silent area usually can be resected without undue morbidity; a similar lesion in the motor strip cannot. A peripheral bronchogenic carcinoma may be cured by surgery while a similar lesion near the tracheal carina cannot be resected. An early carcinoma of the urinary bladder can be cured by limited surgical resection or implantation of radioactive materials; but, when the lesion lies near the bladder trigone, neither of these methods is feasible.

At times, position affects the biologic behavior of the lesion and thereby affects therapy. The chance of lymph node spread varies with position of a lesion within some sites. It is rare to have a lesion which is confined to the vocal cords (glottic larynx) give rise to metastatic adenopathy. In contrast, approximately one-half of all supraglottic larynx lesions are associated with nodal disease. Similarly, lesions of the anterior two-thirds of the tongue have approximately one-half the incidence of nodal metastases associated with lesions of the posterior one-third of the tongue and a considerably lesser incidence of bilateral metastases. Not unpredictably, the cure rate for glottic tumors exceeds that of supraglottic tumors and that of anterior tongue lesions exceeds that of posterior tongue lesions.

Sites of Extension. Every type of tumor at every site has a characteristic mode of growth. For some, local direct infiltration is the prime mechanism. Carcinoma of the cervix is a good example. In others, lymph node metastases occur early and with great frequency. Carcinoma of the nasopharynx behaves in this manner. Last, some tumors give rise to hematogenously-borne distant metastases frequently. Small cell undifferentiated (oat cell) carcinomas of the lung are an example.

These patterns must be considered in treatment planning. To ignore draining lymph nodes in a patient having nasopharyngeal cancer, which presents without clinically evident adenopathy, is to court disaster. On the other hand, to treat clinically negative lymph nodes electively, on the presumption of subclinical involvement, in a patient having a small basal cell carcinoma of the skin, surely is unnecessary.

And yet, the care of every patient must be considered individually. Although therapeutic gains have accrued in some diseases from the administration of "prophylactic" treatment to sites that are likely to have, but cannot be demonstrated to contain tumor, the extent of disease, as best can be detected, is the key to appropriate treatment. As a result, some general rules of management can be formulated for diseases of various extent.

Basic Principles of Treatment: Localized Lesions. In essence, local disease should be treated by local means. Tumors and normal cells are too similar to permit any therapy which acts regionally or systemically to be nearly as effective (with rare exceptions). Moreover, disease which is localized should be curable. This does not mean, however, that anatomic boundaries of treatment should be identical to clinically apparent borders of the lesion. The width of the treatment field should be determined by histologic type, specific site, and morphologic characteristics of the lesion. Because localized therapy, in general, means either surgery or radiotherapy, the previous comments are provided to emphasize the concept that the extent of treatment is dependent on the extent of disease, *not* on the method of treatment. When a given volume must be resected for cure of disease, the same volume must be irradiated for cure and vice versa. If proposed surgical and radiotherapeutic procedures differ in extent, either one method has accepted a risk of underestimating the required volume (because of the inherent morbidity or other limitations of treatment) or the other has overtreated (because of the relative lack of risk of elective treatment). At times these factors can determine which method should be used in a given case. For example, a patient with a small basal cell carcinoma almost surely can be cured by either surgery or radiotherapy. Assuming that the exact size of the lesion is known, treatment of the lesion, including a small margin of surrounding normal tissue, could be accomplished either way. Unfortunately, in clinical practice these lesions may have an indistinct border and a wider margin is necessary to insure inclusion of all disease. If the lesion is situated on the eyelid, the additional morbidity conferred by this margin tends to be greater for surgery than for radiotherapy. In contrast, a basal cell carcinoma of the skin of the trunk usually is better treated by surgery because the abundance of surrounding normal skin permits rapid resection and primary closure without substantial morbidity.

Methods of Localizing Treatment. Radiotherapy can be localized by placing radioactive materials such as radium, radon, iridium, or cesium within a tumor (interstitial therapy), on a body surface directly overlying a tumor (surface mold applicator therapy) or in a natural body cavity adjacent to a tumor (intracavitary therapy). In all three cases, distance between the radioactive source and the tumor is short. Such treatment consequently is known as brachytherapy (brachy meaning short).

Consider a single source of radioactive material. The dose delivered from this source, to any point, depends on three factors: (1) strength of the source, (2) length of time of exposure and (3) the exact distance between source and point. In clinical practice, the first two factors are identical for all tissues concurrently irradiated by a single radioactive source. Thus, the key factor in determining dose is distance and, to be more precise, the dose is a function of the inverse of the distance squared. For example, if in a given time, a source delivers 1,000 rad to a point 1 cm away from itself, at the same time a point 2 cm distant will receive

$$1,000 \times \frac{1}{(2)^2} = 250 \text{ rad}$$

and a point 5 cm distant will receive

$$1,000 \times \frac{1}{(5)^2} = 40 \text{ rad.}$$

Thus, a source implanted in the middle of a 2-cm tumor (1 cm radius) only will inflict 4% $\left(\frac{40}{1,000}\right)$—of the *minimum dose* absorbed by the tumor—upon a normal structure located 5 cm away. Although the exact numbers will differ if more than one source is used or if the source is adjacent to rather than within the tumor, the basic concept remains the same.

If the tumor is in an inaccessible location or, for other reasons, brachytherapy cannot be used, localized treatment can be given by using a beam of poorly penetrating electrons[1] or relatively non-penetrating X or gamma rays.

Basic Principles of Treatment: Regionalized Disease. Regionalized disease potentially is curable but requires treatment of the entire tumor including the most distant sites of extension and intervening tissues *en bloc*. Disease which has a high likelihood of spread to lymph nodes falls into this category, even if *proof* of regionalization has not been obtained. (Tumors which have spread to nodes but also have disseminated widely should *not* be treated in this fashion; if they are to be cured, they require systemic therapy.)

An example of regional therapy likely to come to mind is surgical—the classical radical mastectomy including axillary lymph node dissection. In this procedure, the breast primary, surrounding tissues and potentially involved axillary lymph nodes are removed concurrently, in one piece. However, the procedure is not a perfect example, because it leaves the internal mammary nodes untreated and they represent a likely site of spread particularly with medially or centrally located primary tumors. Actually, radiotherapeutic management of early breast cancer (Chap. 2) provides a better example, because all of the potentially involved nodal stations are treated. In fact, radiotherapy has its greatest therapeutic advantage in the treatment of regionalized disease. Consider another example, a tumor of the base of the tongue.

Overall, approximately 80% of such lesions will give rise to cervical lymph node metastases, and of these, a substantial proportion will be bilateral even when lymphatic disease is not grossly evident. Basic principles dictate that treatment include both sides of the neck even when they appear uninvolved. In reality, however, when surgery is employed for such tumors, this is not always done because morbidity of bilateral neck dissections—either concomitant or metachronous—is considerable. Thus, a modified (or in some way limited) procedure sometimes is advocated for one side of the neck. At times only a unilateral dissection is done on the side the surgeon believes to be at greater risk. These procedures balance the *possibility* of disease recurrence against the *certain* morbidity of the surgical procedure. In contrast, bilateral neck irradiation to doses which sterilize subclinical disease in the overwhelming majority of cases, is well tolerated and presents no compromise.

Methods of Regionalizing Therapy. The most common methods of radiotherapy are well suited to treating regional disease. In essence, these methods use x rays (generated electronically) or gamma rays (generated by disintegration of radioactive elements) from sources relatively distant from tumors (teletherapy). This permits large fields to be irradiated homogeneously. In addition, it permits treatment of lesions located at relatively great depths below the skin surface.

Occasionally, chemotherapy is used in a regional manner. By selectively infusing drug into tumor or by restricting drugs' ability to dissipate by continually perfusing it through an area (Chap. 11), regionalized therapy is effected.

Basic Principles of Treatment: Disseminated Disease. Disseminated disease implies hematogenous spread and in most instances incurability. In general, this is equally true for the patient who has 1 metastatic lesion and the patient who has 100 metastatic lesions. Once a metastatic lesion appears, others are likely to follow. As a result, the aim of treatment for such patients should primarily be focused on improving or protecting the *quality* of life and only secondarily, if possible, extending its duration. In our opinion, it is senseless to trade 6 months of comfortable productive life for 7 months of discomfort.

Methods of Systemic Therapy. Systemic therapy is nearly synonymous with chemotherapy. It is in this forum that chemotherapy has proven itself to be one of the three *established* methods of cancer treatment. Depending on the pharmacology of the drug(s) being used, oral, intramuscular or intravenous administration routes all result in systemic distribution and action.

Radiotherapy also can be used as systemic therapy in certain circumstances. For radiosensitive diseases, such as chronic lymphocytic leukemia or lymphocytic lymphomas, low dose, whole body radiotherapy can provide an alternative to chemotherapy.[2,3] With less sensitive disease, single fraction, large dose, half-body irradiation is becoming a proven method of achieving palliation.[1]

In addition, it should be remembered that, at times, the best systemic therapy consists solely of supportive care. A patient who has widely disseminated squamous cell bronchogenic carcinoma which is asymptomatic and does not imminently threaten any vital structure, probably should *not* be given either chemotherapy or radiotherapy except in a well-controlled experimental trial. No known regimen will significantly alter his or her prognosis, and since the patient is asymptomatic, no regimen can improve the quality of his or her life. One should *never* treat solely on the basis of a positive scan, x ray or laboratory report; always treat on the basis of the patient's needs. Moreover, even if the patient becomes symptomatic, *systemic* therapy is not indicated automatically. Diffuse minor aches and pains can often be treated more effectively by analgesics than by antitumor therapy. When one metastatic site is particularly painful, local palliative therapy to that site alone, can be dramatically effective.

Effect of Specific Site on Treatment. In addition to spatial relationship of sites being a key factor in treatment, certain sites in and of themselves are important determinants of therapy. Some sites preclude treatment by one or another means. Vital structures cannot be resected. Tumors involving some areas of brain, or both lobes of the liver or trachea, in essence, cannot be treated surgically. Anatomic regions which provide essential structural support also cannot be resected. Cervical vertebral bodies or the base of the skull are examples.

Similarly, curative radiotherapy is ill advised in organs which have normal cells that are relatively sensitive to irradiation. In such cases irradiation doses required for permanent control of disease may either destroy an essential function or induce intolerable complications. Cancers residing in the liver or stomach are examples of tumors which are rarely treated for cure by radiotherapy because of these problems.

Partially because drugs are rarely used as the sole method of treatment for cure of solid tumors and partially because drugs act systemically in most cases, previously discussed factors are not primary concerns in chemotherapeutic management. On the other hand, certain sites do protect tumors from the action of chemotherapy. Central nervous system metastases are shielded from chemotherapeutic action. In fact, one of the major problems currently encountered in treatment of chemosensitive tumors is the relatively high failure rate secondary to brain metastases. For example, if particular attention is not directed toward treatment of this region, approximately one-half of all first relapses in children, having acute lymphocytic leukemia, will be in the central nervous system.[5] Precisely, why this should occur is unclear. Often this pattern is attributed to inability of the drug to cross from blood into brain because of the so-called "blood brain barrier." But there is no "blood *tumor* barrier." In fact, routinely we rely on the ability of a radioisotope to cross from blood into the area of a brain tumor for detection on a scan.

A second, but less common, site of protection occurs in the testes. Failure at this site occasionally is a problem in acute leukemia but again the explanation is unclear.

In addition, the site to which disease has metastasized appears to affect the ability of specific drugs to act upon the tumor at that site. For example, cyclophosphamide, methotrexate and 5-fluorouracil have become a relatively standard combination of drugs which is effective against breast cancer. However, Greenspan[6] notes that each drug, by itself, has greater or lesser activity than the others at some sites. Cyclophosphamide is particularly active against metastatic pulmonary or diffuse osseous disease; methotrexate against metastatic skin or subcutaneous disease and 5-fluorouracil against intra-abdominal disease. Why the same tumor should be more or less sensitive to different drugs when it metastasizes to various sites, remains to be explained.

Effect of Site on Timing of Treatment. In general, treatment should be based on extent and type of disease and, within reason, as much time as is required to complete a metastatic work-up should be allowed prior to therapy; however, disease involving certain sites forces the oncologist to treat with dispatch. At times, treatment must be rapid, at others urgent.

In effect, the need for rapid therapy in certain circumstances precludes the use of hormones at those times. For example, a postmenopausal woman who has carcinoma of the breast metastatic to several subcutaneous sites, is a suitable candidate for estrogen therapy because she can afford to wait up to 8 weeks for response. However, if this woman also has pulmonary lymphangitic spread or diffuse hepatic metastases, treatment must be designed to produce a rapid antitumor effect, and cytotoxic drugs, rather than hormones, are required. At other sites treatment must be given within 24 to 48 hours, even if work-up is incomplete or a tissue diagnosis is not available.

Emergency Therapy. Two anatomic regions, chest and central nervous system, when invaded by tumor, may demand emergency treatment. Within the chest, obstruction of blood flow to the heart through the superior vena cava is potentially fatal. While less dramatic, epidural metastases which compress spinal cord can produce permanent paraparesis or paraplegia if not treated before damage becomes irreversible. Thus, these presentations require treatment almost immediately.

Superior vena caval obstruction results in a syndrome of facial swelling and edema, plethora or cyanosis, dyspnea and distention of the collateral venous circulation of the neck and thorax. In nearly all instances, the syndrome is secondary to tumor. Perez et al.[7] in their review of the subject, noted that benign etiologies account for only 3% of the syndrome as compared with bronchogenic carcinomas which account for approximately 80% of cases and lymphomas accounting for an additional 10%. (However, the syndrome is uncommon, occurring in only approximately 5% of all bronchogenic carcinomas.) Treatment must be given without delay and histologic confirmation of tumor in this circumstance is not mandatory.

Radiotherapy forms the mainstay of treatment and in expert hands[7] yields symptomatic relief in 70% of cases caused by carcinoma (20% complete relief, 50% partial relief) and in 95% of cases caused by malignant lymphoma (75% complete relief, 20% partial relief). Chemotherapy sometimes is used as an adjuvant to irradiation but its precise role is unclear.

Spinal cord compression initially presents as back pain but usually has progressed to produce motor loss before diagnosis. If untreated, sensory loss followed by loss of sphincter control in advanced cases will occur. Although any type of tumor can produce these symptoms, one-half of all cases result from bronchogenic carcinomas, lymphomas or tumors without a detectable primary site.[8]

Appropriate therapy must be directed toward precise sites of disease. Statistically, approximately 70% of cases occur in the thoracic spinal cord. Motor or sensory dermatome levels and x-ray films of the spine may localize position of the lesion. However, the *sine qua non* for localization is a myelogram which will demonstrate the superior and inferior limits of the gross lesion and may detect additional lesions which are clinically silent.

Appropriate therapy varies with histologic type of causative tumor, duration of the block, anatomic level of the lesion and overall physical condition of the patient. As an initial temporizing measure, the anti-inflammatory effect of corticosteroids appears to be of value. Next, histologic cell type should be determined; if no known primary tumor can be found, laminectomy should be done to establish the diagnosis, help plan subsequent therapy and simultaneously provide decompression. When histologic type can be predicted on the basis of pre-existing disease, laminectomy can still provide rapid decompression for rapid, progressive disease, particularly for tumors which are un-likely to respond quickly to irradiation. On the other hand, for radiosensitive disease, such as lymphoma or multiple myeloma, rapid institution of irradiation as the sole treatment will suffice[8] and will eliminate the uncommon but potentially dire risks of laminectomy. Gilbert et al.[9] have compared results of radiation therapy vs. laminectomy plus radiation in a large number of patients and found no difference in outcome. Laminectomy is therefore not used generally for patients having long standing compression, for patients in poor general medical condition and for lesions at the level of the cauda equina.

Prognosis depends upon pretreatment status of the patient and histologic type of the tumor. Bruckman and Bloomer[8] note that 60% of patients who are ambulatory at diagnosis remain ambulatory, while only 7% of patients who are paraplegic at diagnosis recover sufficiently to ambulate. When histologic cell type is considered, a distinct advantage is seen for patients who have relatively radiosensitive tumors. Approximately 50% of such patients remain or become ambulatory as compared to approximately 10% of patients having less responsive lesions such as kidney tumors.

Effect of Site on Prognosis. The involvement by tumor of a vital structure can radically decrease survival. On the other hand, disease literally can destroy a non-vital site without substantially affecting prognosis. Consequently, once a tumor has metastasized, the precise nature of afflicted organs becomes as important in determining prognosis, if not more so, than basic biologic behavior of the disease. For example, Pearlman and Jochimsen[10] reviewed the survival of women who had recurrent breast cancer. When the initial site of recurrence was in bone or soft tissue, patients fared best, exhibiting a median survival of 22 to 26 months. In cases where the first recurrence was in pleura or lung, median survival was 10 to 12 months and when disease first recurred as liver or brain metastases, survival dropped to 4 to 6 months. In fact, the site of disease governed prognosis far more than did the choice of initial therapy for the recurrence.

Alternatively, the same conclusions can be drawn by examining the prognosis of patients having different types of tumors which have metastasized to the same vital organ. When this is done, the conclusion that the effect of site of metastatic disease outweighs individuality of the disease which has metastasized to it, is inescapable. For example, Hendrickson[11] reported the Radiation Therapy Oncology Group's data from a trial of palliative whole brain irradiation for different types of cerebral metastases. Patients were grouped by anatomic site of their primary disease and classified by severity of their neurologic findings. When pre-treatment and post-treatment status were compared, the maximum difference between lung tumors, breast tumors or all other tumors, in terms of the percentage of patients who improved, stayed stable or deteriorated, was *less than 3%*. Similarly, survival of patients who have brain metastases is nearly identical independent of site of origin.[12]

References

1. Tapley, N. duV., (ed.): *Clinical Applications of the Electron Beam*. New York, John Wiley and Sons, 1976.
2. Johnson, R.E. and Ruhl, U.: Treatment of Chronic Lymphocytic Leukemia with Emphasis on Total Body Irradiation. Int. J. Radiat. Oncol., Biol., Phys. *1*:387–397, 1976.
3. Chaffey, J.T., et al.: Advanced Lymphosarcoma Treated by Total Body Irradiation. Br. J. Cancer *31*:441–449, 1975.
4. Fitzpatrick, P.J. and Rider, W.D.: Half Body Radiotherapy. Int. J. Radiat. Oncol., Biol., Phys. *1*:197–207, 1976.
5. Pinkel, D., et al.: Radiotherapy in Leukemia and Lymphoma of Children. Cancer *39*:817–824, 1977.
6. Greenspan, E.M.: Breast Cancer. In, *Clinical Cancer Chemotherapy*, ed. Greenspan, E.M., New York, Raven Press, 1975.
7. Perez, C.A., Presant, C.A. and VanAmburg, A.L.: Management of Superior Vena Cava Syndrome. Semin. Oncol. *5*:123–134, 1978.
8. Bruckman, J.E. and Bloomer, W.D.: Management of Spinal Cord Compression. Semin. Oncol. *5*:135–140, 1978.
9. Gilbert, H., et al.: Neoplastic Epidural Spinal Cord Compression. J.A.M.A. *240*:2771–2773, 1978.
10. Pearlman, N.W. and Jochimsen, P.R.: Recurrent Breast Cancer: Factors Influencing Survival, Including Treatment. J. Surg. Oncol. *11*:21–29, 1979.
11. Hendrickson, F.R.: Radiation Therapy of Metastatic Tumors. Semin. Oncol. *2*:43–46, 1975.
12. Nisce, L.Z., Hilaris, B.S. and Chu, F.C.H.: A Review of Experience with Irradiation of Brain Metastases. A.J.R. *111*:329–333, 1971.

THE
RATIONALE

The
Host

(

13
EFFECT OF
AGE AND SEX

Although cancers commonly are viewed as unregulated growths, there is abundant evidence to the contrary. Cancers appear to have internal structure (Chap. 9), and the growth of many cancers is regulated by available oxygen and nutrient (Chap. 11). In addition, various factors associated with the host may relate to the probability of occurrence of specific cancers. For example, certain cancers display a familial pattern; persons with close relatives having a particular cancer have a greater risk of contracting that type of cancer than do others having no close relatives with the disease. Persons having certain genetic diseases (such as xeroderma pigmentosa or Fanconi's anemia) have incidences of cancer much higher than does the population at large. Thus host status clearly may influence tumor growth. The purpose of this chapter is to examine the effect of the host's age and sex on the likelihood of cancer occurrence and thereafter in its management.

Effect of Age Upon Tumor Type. There can be little question that a person's age significantly influences his likelihood of developing a tumor, and more specifically, a particular type of tumor. Tumors occur only rarely in young adulthood and are unusual in childhood, but arise frequently in the elderly. Practically speaking, some tumors occur only during certain age ranges. Neuroblastomas, Wilms' tumors, and acute lymphoblastic leukemia, for example, occur almost entirely in children. Ewing's sarcoma rarely occurs in other than adolescents. Other tumors, while most common in certain age groups, have a wider age range of occurrence. Ovarian tumors are most frequent in patients beyond middle age; however, they are not rare in women even as young as their twenties. Still other types of tumors have bi-modal age distributions. Hodgkin's disease occurs primarily in late adolescence and early adulthood but has a second peak of incidence in persons in their fifties. Similarly, non-Hodgkin's lymphomas on the whole affect children and the elderly, generally sparing young adults and persons who are middle aged. In fact, every tumor has a characteristic age distribution. As a result, the type of cancer commonly seen is highly dependent upon the age group of patients studied. As can be seen from Table 13–1, which lists the most common types of fatal cancers in various age ranges, the host significantly influences the types of cancer which the physician is likely to encounter.

In an analogous manner, the sex of the host substantially affects the type of cancers that form. Of course, cancer cannot arise from non-existent organs. Consequently, carcinomas of prostate, cervix, endometrium and ovary are sex specific. The incidence of other tumors,

Table 13–1.   Cancers Which Produce Greatest Mortality by Age and Sex

Age	Male	Female
under 15	1. Leukemia 2. Brain and Nervous Tissue 3. Bone 4. Kidney 5. Connective Tissue	1. Leukemia 2. Brain and Nervous Tissue 3. Kidney 4. Bone 5. Connective Tissue
15–34	1. Leukemia 2. Brain and Nervous Tissue 3. Testis 4. Hodgkin's Disease 5. Skin	1. Leukemia 2. Breast 3. Brain and Nervous Tissue 4. Uterus 5. Hodgkin's Disease
35–54	1. Lung 2. Colon and Rectum 3. Pancreas 4. Brain and Nervous Tissue 5. Leukemia	1. Breast 2. Lung 3. Colon and Rectum 4. Uterus 5. Ovary
55–75	1. Lung 2. Colon and Rectum 3. Prostate 4. Pancreas 5. Stomach	1. Breast 2. Colon and Rectum 3. Lung 4. Ovary 5. Uterus
over 75	1. Lung 2. Prostate 3. Colon and Rectum 4. Stomach 5. Bladder	1. Colon and Rectum 2. Breast 3. Lung 4. Pancreas 5. Uterus

however, also correlates highly with the host's sex. Carcinoma of the breast is 100 times as common in females as in males, and head and neck cancer is overwhelmingly a disease of men. Precisely why this should occur is unclear. Perhaps the frequency of breast cancer in women is related to the greater exposure of their breasts to estrogenic stimulation (see promotional stimulus for cancer growth—Chap. 1). Perhaps the dominance in men of head and neck cancers relates to their more frequent abuse of alcohol and tobacco, causative factors in the induction of cancers (Chap. 1). However, these factors probably account for only part of the picture because, for example, carcinomas of the post-cricoid hypopharynx occur frequently in women. Still other tumors are common in both sexes. Carcinomas of the colon and rectum are an example.

Effect Upon Site of Disease. The anatomic sites likely to be affected by tumors vary with the host's age in two ways. For the many types of tumors that only can arise in one organ, the likelihood of involvement of that site varies according to that tumor's frequency in each age group. Because every tumor tends to spread in a characteristic fashion, the probability of involvement of other organs, which are frequent sites of metastatic spread, follows a similar pattern. For tumors that can arise in more than one organ, for example, lymphomas, and tumors that can arise at different sites with a given organ, for example, brain tumors, the host's age can affect the precise site of disease. Non-Hodgkin's lymphomas in children occur within the gastrointestinal tract in approximately one-third of cases. In contrast, non-Hodgkin's lymphoma in the elderly uncommonly arises in these sites. Primary brain tumors in adults occur in the cerebral hemispheres almost exclusively. In contrast, infra-tentorial brain tumors predominate in children.

Effect Upon Histologic Type. In anatomic sites which frequently give rise to tumors of varying histology, age of the host substantially influences the cell type of tumor likely to arise. Ovarian tumors in children tend to be derivatives of granulosa or theca cell lines and may lead to precocious or aberrant sexual development. Ovarian tumors in adolescence and early adulthood tend to be teratomas. Ovarian cancers, in older women, arise from cells of the surface epithelium, and usually are serous cystadenocarcinomas, mucinous cystadenocarcinomas or endometroid cystadenocarcinomas. Similarly, thyroid carcinomas in the young, tend to be papillary; follicular tumors become common in middle age and anaplastic tumors basically are restricted to the elderly. In fact, even within one histologic type, the degree of differentiation varies with age. Brain tumors in children frequently are well-differentiated, cystic types, while glioblastoma multiforme is the predominant brain tumor in adults. Patients in their twenties tend to have the nodular sclerosing variant of Hodgkin's disease, while elderly patients tend to have mixed cellular and lymphocyte depletion disease.

To some extent, the host's sex also affects degree of differentiation. With either primary brain tumors or Hodgkin's disease, females tend to have better differentiated tumors and therefore better prognosis.

Effect of Age Upon Clinical Presentation. Odd as it may seem, the age of the patient may influence the manner in which a tumor presents itself. Neuroblastomas provide a good example. Babies under 2 years old usually are found to have neuroblastomas when a mass, representing the primary tumor, is palpated in the abdomen. In other respects the child appears well. However, children over the age of 2 usually are found to have a neuroblastoma only after the lesion has given rise to osseous metastases which are painful. Such children manifest discomfort and are irritable and restless, not at all like their younger counterparts.

Effect of Age Upon Management. The age of the host influences treatment in a number of ways. In addition to the previously described effects upon the tumor itself, age of the host significantly can alter management. Tolerance to treatment is inseparably related to age. Growing children must be treated cautiously to avoid iatrogenic short stature or scoliosis whenever possible. In fact, most radiotherapists prescribe pediatric doses on a sliding scale, depending upon the patient's age. There is some evidence to indicate that tumors in young children are relatively sensitive to treatment; however, the known toxicity of treatment in young children is the basic deciding factor necessitating lesser doses of radiation than are commonly administered to adults. On the other hand, when chemotherapeutic doses are compared on a per kilogram body weight or per square meter of surface area basis, children tolerate relatively greater doses than adults.

Treatment may need to be modified to deal with tumors in persons who are sexually potent and wish to bear children. While the desire to maintain reproductive potential cannot outweigh necessity of therapy, in those instances where alternatives or modifications of therapy preserve sexual potency, great pains should be taken to see that this is done. For example, treatment of infradiaphragmatic Hodgkin's disease must include the lymph node chains in the pelvis. When males are treated by radiotherapy, meticulous collimation of radiation ports and specific shielding of testes preserves fertility. If females were irradiated in the same manner, the ovaries would be within irradiated fields. Consequently, as part of the staging laparotomy, routine oophoropexy, moving the ovaries out of the irradiated field, should be done. Many females who are treated in this manner maintain normal menstrual function and several normal healthy children have been born to women so treated and cured of disease. In contrast, patients who have advanced Hodgkin's disease must be treated by chemotherapy. Because it is not possible to shield reproductive organs from the effects of the drugs, infertility in males occurs routinely.

Age also may modify management because of patients' inability to cooperate. This is most apparent in children who do not understand the nature of their disease or the necessity of treatment. In particular, for a procedure such as radiotherapy, where patient cooperation is vital for accurate positioning, sedation and sometimes anesthesia must be added to whatever regimen is otherwise necessary to insure adequate therapy. In turn, because of the hazards of repetitive anesthesia, prolonged courses of treatment are not practical. For similar reasons, chemotherapy in children is best done with non-oral medicines to obviate the need for patient cooperation in swallowing.

Although advanced age *per se* is not a contraindication to treatment, one must also modify treatment in deference to advanced age. Elderly patients do not tolerate aggressive multidrug chemotherapeutic regimens tolerated by younger patients. In addition, shorter survival of such patients may permit less aggressive therapy which, nevertheless, keeps the patient relatively free of the effects of disease for the rest of his or her survival.

Effect of Age Upon Complications of Treatment. The age at which a person receives non-surgical therapy for cancer influences the likelihood of subsequent complications. As already described, elderly patients tolerate treatment poorly and acute reactions to treatment are generally worse for them. However, for those patients who can be taken through therapy, both young and old patients may experience complications, although their explanations may differ. It is easy to understand how elderly patients who are treated by radiotherapy for carcinoma of the cervix tend to have complications which can be explained on the basis of their less distensible tissues and consequent less than optimum placement of intracavitary applicators, resulting in less than optimum dose. Far less understandable is the increased rate of complications in patients who are treated in their thirties when compared to the average patient in her fifties. Why this should be so is unclear; however, it is a fact. Last, as will be discussed in Chapter 19, a feared complication of treatment is the induction of a second neoplasm. While the overall risk of this happening is small, the risk of cancer induction in patients who are treated in childhood is considerably greater than in those patients who are treated as adults.

Effect Upon Prognosis. For reasons that remain only partly understood, the age at which a patient develops a neoplasm may affect that patient's prognosis. Neuroblastomas in young children sometimes spontaneously will transform into benign ganglioneuromas. For other diseases, advancing age may be associated with more poorly differentiated types of tumors. As discussed in Chapter 6, the degree of differentiation affects both therapy and prognosis and in this indirect manner, age affects therapy and prognosis. However, the affect of age upon prognosis cannot be explained on this basis for other tumors. Children who are afflicted by acute lymphocytic leukemia toward the end of the first decade of life, in general, fare much worse than those who are afflicted around age 3.

Sexual factors also affect prognosis. For a number of diseases, for example, Hodgkin's lymphoma and malignant melanoma, females fare better than males.

Effect Upon Interpretation. A key objective in oncology, as in medicine in general, is to improve continually the quality of care. Among the many yardsticks used to measure success of therapy, survival frequently is viewed as the most important. However, survival is highly dependent upon the patient's age at the time of discovery of disease. If it were possible, for example, to ensure that treatment of testicular carcinoma and prostatic carcinoma were in every respect equally successful, crude survival rate from testicular carcinoma would always exceed that of prostatic carcinoma. In the normal course of events patients in the prostatic cancer group would be ravaged by a large variety of other ills (because of their advanced age) to which testicular carcinoma patients (who, on the whole, are young) would not be subject. Thus as has already been discussed in Chapter 4, when one wishes to compare two populations of dissimilar age, it is essential to use relative survival data to compensate for deaths due to other causes.

14

INTENTION OF
TREATMENT

All therapy should have a specific *purpose* and this purpose should influence the manner in which therapy is administered. Although this interrelationship is crucial, in practice, not infrequently, one part of the relationship seems to overshadow the other. The patient's main question is "what can be done for me?" The referring physician asks "what is the patient's prognosis?" The oncologist primarily must be concerned with the possible benefits of treatment. And yet, it is the *"nuts and bolts"* of therapy that the patient must endure, the referring physician must agree to, and the oncologist must prescribe. The purpose of this chapter is to explore the mechanisms of therapy in terms of their dependence upon the intention of treatment.

Intentions of Treatment. Four basic objectives justify treatment: (1) cure of disease, (2) palliation of symptoms, (3) prevention of impending signs or symptoms and (4) prolongation of useful life. Each of these objectives is of value to the patient, however, not of equal value. Thus, logical management must balance adverse aspects against potential benefits of therapy.

Cure of disease obviously is the most desirable outcome of therapy. It permits the patient to resume interrupted plans and live a "normal" lifespan. And, it eliminates need for future therapy.

In general, cure comes about when *localized* disease is controlled by local means. Actually, *local control* of disease is all that can be asked of local therapy. However, if work-up has excluded detectable distant metastases and undetectable distant metastases are absent, cure is an outgrowth of local control.

The precise criteria of cure or local control vary with the type of tumor. In general, if disease has not recurred within 5 years the patient is considered cured. However, this concept is somewhat inadequate. Some tumors either recur quickly or not at all. Nearly all recurrences after treatment of tumors arising in head and neck sites (excluding true vocal cord lesions) are evident within 3 years. For most pediatric tumors, Collins' law[1] applies. The period of risk of recurrence is approximately equal to the patient's age when the tumor is diagnosed plus 9 months (the maximum time the tumor could have existed in utero). In contrast, there is risk of recurrence of other types of tumors for many years after therapy. Benign tumors, low grade brain tumors and thyroid tumors frequently recur more than 5 years after diagnosis and treatment. Distant metastases which are first seen 10 years after treatment of localized breast cancer are not rare. Yet, most *local recurrences* of breast cancer do occur within 2 years of treatment.

For non-solid neoplasms, the concept of localized disease must be modified. Some non-Hodgkin's lymphomas occur as localized disease in non-nodal sites. Early Hodgkin's disease, occurring in one site, represents localized disease. Solitary plasmacytomas represent *localized* multiple myeloma but other tumors, such as the leukemias, do not have a localized phase. In these cases equivalent factors, for example, an almost normal blood count, indicate earlier disease. In any case, cure generally is accepted when no evidence of disease is found after 5 years. In contrast with solid tumors, local and systemic means can bring about prolonged disease-free survival in some situations. And unlike solid tumors, advanced, disseminated disease can be treated with this intention.

Palliation of Symptoms. When cure is not a realistic possibility, amelioration of distressing signs or symptoms which prevent the patient from fully utilizing his remaining life, becomes of paramount importance.

While it is not possible to define all situations for which palliative therapy is beneficial, the following should serve to provide a representative sample. Painful metastases (usually osseous), bronchial obstruction producing post-obstructive pneumonia, cough or hemoptysis secondary to pulmonary tumors, neurologic signs and symptoms secondary to brain metastases, superior vena caval obstruction and spinal cord compression are just some situations that frequently benefit from palliative treatment.

Prophylactic Therapy/Prolongation of Life. When cure is not possible and the patient is asymptomatic, a strong case can be made for not upsetting the patient by administering any aggressive therapy—with some important exceptions. These exceptions concern the patient who has a tumor which is highly likely to become a substantial management problem in the near future—or for which therapy is available which will significantly increase projected survival.

Prophylactic therapy means different things to different people. To some, treatment aimed at "growth restraint" is justified. In general, we do not agree unless such therapy will likely lengthen patients' survival and can be effected with little morbidity. Merely improving the findings of a patient's x-ray film does not necessarily translate into improved medical care. Effecting "growth restraint" of a non-threatening cutaneous lesion is without merit if the patient is dying of hepatic metastases. On the other hand, when a patient (1) has more than a few weeks to live, (2) has a lesion that is in imminent risk of producing distressing symptoms which will require therapy and which will decrease the quality of the patient's survival, and (3) would have symptoms which can be prevented by *less* toxic therapy, prophylactic treatment is warranted. Examples of such situations include a right upper lobe bronchogenic carcinoma that is beginning to compress the vena cava, a chest wall recurrence from a breast cancer which is about to ulcerate or hemorrhage, or an epidural metastases which has been decompressed surgically and is asymptomatic but surely will regrow in the near future.

The other major exception to the rule of thumb, "no cure, no symptoms, no treatment" concerns those situations wherein a substantial increase in proleptic, useful survival can be produced at reasonable cost. Of course, what is reasonable can be debated, but the general principle should be clear. Examples that justify such treatment include chemotherapeutic management of advanced ovarian carcinoma or advanced oat cell bronchogenic carcinoma.

Risks and Side Effects. Once an assessment of the possible objectives of treatment has been completed, the oncologist must consider risks involved in methods capable of achieving these goals. If cure of disease is possible, a substantial incidence of temporary, adverse reactions during therapy can be tolerated. A small incidence of severe complications can be justified, if patients can be cured. However, if palliation of distressing symptoms is the aim, there is no benefit in exchanging equally unpleasant side effects of therapy for unpleasant effects of disease. Moreover, it is unconscionable to inflict complications in addition to the patient's disease. Similarly, when prevention of future symptoms is the object, neither side effects nor complications are acceptable. Treatment aimed at prolonging life must be individualized—if the length of prolongation markedly exceeds the duration of the reactions associated with treatment, it is likely to be acceptable. Minor complications too, may be tolerated, but major ones may not.

Duration of Therapy. Unlike that of surgery, the duration of radiotherapy ranges from days to weeks and that of chemotherapy from months to years. If the patient can be cured of disease and returned to active life, such protracted treatment can be justified. Similarly, if substantial prolongation of life is possible, intermittent therapy over a considerable span, so long as it does not occupy the bulk of the patient's time, is warranted. On the other hand, when palliation or prophylaxis is the goal, the quickest, least distressing means of achieving this end should be sought.

Dose and Complexity. In general, the minimum dose that will sterilize a tumor depends upon that tumor, but the maximum dose that can be given to a tumor depends upon the tolerance of simultaneously affected normal tissues. With chemotherapy, other than changing the dose or regionalizing the effects (Chap. 11), the amount delivered to tumor or normal tissues is relatively fixed. On the other hand, one of the prime advantages of modern high energy radiotherapy equipment is the ability to deliver radiation to precisely localized volumes. Coupled with computerized treatment planning, nearly any desired volume can be homogeneously irradiated and any other region spared. When cure of disease is the objective, doses approaching normal tissue tolerance often are necessary and the time, expense and difficulty inherent in complex treatment planning prove to be an excellent investment. In contrast, when palliation or prevention is the aim, a decrease in the volume of disease, rather than complete eradication, is all that is necessary. Consequently, lesser doses can and should be used, i.e. doses well below tolerance levels. As a result, simple plans which can be quickly, inexpensively and easily constructed become the preferred form of treatment. Some important exceptions to this rule exist. Certain tumors, in particular neoplasms arising in the head and neck region, simply do not respond to the lesser doses which produce palliation of other types of tumors. When such lesions are treated for palliation, moderately high doses and moderately complex treatment plans become necessary.

The Tumor. A main theme throughout this book describes the individuality of different types of cancers and this individuality also influences the way in which therapy should be delivered. One must consider the likely course of untreated or sub-aggressively treated disease. For example, different grade primary brain tumors behave substantially differently. Anaplastic tumors uniformly are fatal within a few months, while well-differentiated tumors are compatible with years of useful life. Highly aggressive radiotherapy of glioblastomas has helped to prolong the life of affected patients—therapy that likely would produce an unacceptable incidence of complications were the patients to have substantial subsequent survival. In contrast, patients who have well-differentiated astrocytomas, live long enough to manifest complications, were they treated in the same manner, and when radiotherapy is administered for such disease, it should be given in a less aggressive fashion.

The same concept also applies to chemotherapeutic management. For some diseases, such as chronic lymphocytic leukemia, gentle intermittent therapy can yield years of useful life. When disease progresses, reinstitution or escalation of therapy frequently produces another remission. On the other hand, some diseases not only relapse rapidly, but once relapse occurs, a second remission can be induced only rarely. Diffuse histiocytic lymphoma is an example. The individual differences between even similar diseases can be great. Merely within the category of non-Hodgkin's lymphoma, the difference between diffuse histiocytic disease and nodular lymphocytic disease, which relapses slowly and frequently can be forced back into remission, is striking. Therapy of the former must be aggressive, but does produce some long term survivors, while therapy of the latter can be less toxic and still be effective. Treatment of diffuse histiocytic lymphomas must be aimed at producing a *complete* response. Partial regression seems not to produce any appreciable benefit. In contrast, treatment of nodular lymphocytic lymphomas can rely on subsequent management to be beneficial and ultra-aggressive regimens need not be used for initial therapy.

Is Treatment Appropriate? The decision to administer or withhold therapy needs be considered carefully. It not only should be based upon type and extent of disease, but also upon an assessment of the patient's overall condition. When the patient's general condition is good, any of the previously discussed concepts can apply. However, when the patient's condition is poor, treatment may have to be altered or even deferred. Even if the extent and type of neoplastic disease potentially can be cured, the patient must be able to withstand therapy. Non-neoplastic disease that precludes aggressive management, contraindicates radical treatment as effectively as disseminated neoplastic disease. In such situations, the discussions referrable to palliative therapy are more germane to that patient's care than those concerning curative therapy. When the patient's condition is extremely poor, even gentle palliative therapy may not be warranted.

Table 14–1.   Karnofsky Criteria of Performance Status (PS)

Able to Carry on Normal Activity; No Special Care is Needed	100%	Normal; no complaints; no evidence of disease.
	90%	Able to carry on normal activity; minor signs or symptoms of disease.
	80%	Normal activity with effort; some signs or symptoms of disease.
Unable to Work; Able to Live at Home; Cares for Most Personal Needs; A Varying Amount of Assistance is Needed	70%	Cares for self; unable to carry on normal activity or to do active work.
	60%	Requires occasional assistance but is able to care for most of his needs.
	50%	Requires considerable assistance and frequent medical care.
Unable to Care for Self; Requires Equivalent of Institutional or Hospital Care; Disease may be Progressing Rapidly	40%	Disabled; requires special medical care and assistance.
	30%	Severely disabled; hospitalization is indicated, although death not imminent.
	20%	Very sick; hospitalization necessary; active supportive treatment necessary.
	10%	Moribund; fatal processes progressing rapidly.
	0%	Dead.

Table 14–2.   Eastern Cooperative Oncology Group—Zubrod Criteria of Performance Status (PS)

0—No symptoms; normal activity
1—Symptoms, fully ambulatory
2—Needs to be in bed <50% of day
3—Needs to be in bed >50% of day
4—Unable to get out of bed

Host Factors. Just as the status of the tumor can be quantified by staging (Chap. 3), the overall condition of the host can be designated by a numerical grade. Two systems are in common use and the rules governing category assignment in each are listed in Tables 14–1 and 2. As can be seen, they differ mainly in the degree of grouping or separation. In either system, criteria are independent of type or extent of tumor and can (and should) be used not only prior to therapy, but repeatedly, as part of routine follow-up care.

Reference

1. Collins, V.P.: The Treatment of Wilms' Tumor. Cancer *11*:89–94, 1958.

15

INDIRECT EFFECTS

Most, if not all cancers, produce effects at sites distant from those they occupy. While cancers physically may be confined, their effects can involve the entire body and often the mind as well. In this sense, even local or regional disease can be viewed as systemic. The mechanisms by which this occurs vary, and may involve mechanical, pharmacological, nutritional or psychiatric pathways, and there may well be some which are as yet unknown.

Mechanical Distant Effects. Occasionally, distant effects may be observed when a cancer compromises the function of an organ in which it is growing. If other organs depend on the impaired organ, their function may be impaired as well. An example of such a situation occurs in some patients who have lung cancer. When pulmonary function is sufficiently reduced by cancer, other parts of the body may suffer from hypoxia and both structural and functional changes are observed. By virtue of its location, a lung tumor may compress the vena cava (Chap. 12) and impede return of blood to the heart. In turn, a relative deficit in cardiac output and a more obvious back-up of blood flow in the vessels which feed into the vena cava ensues. These changes manifest systemically as altered venous drainage patterns (collateral circulation), increased intravenous pressure within head and neck vessels, cyanosis and dyspnea.

In a somewhat analogous manner, an intracerebral tumor which locally produces increased pressure will manifest distantly as projectile vomiting. Another example is the relationship between renal tumors and hypertension. While some kidney cancers secrete sub-

197

stances that increase blood pressure, others seem to do so simply by increasing intracapsular tension.

Pharmacologic Effects. Some tumors produce distant effects by liberating pharmacologically active substances. They may be by-products or excretory products of tumor metabolism, but nevertheless are synthesized by particular cancers. An exhaustive list of such substances is beyond the scope of this book, but several general categories and examples of the paraneoplastic effects they produce are provided to illustrate the point.

Hormone Secretion. Some cancers of endocrine glands continue to secrete the type of hormone produced by the gland from which they arose. Thyroid carcinoma may secrete thyroid hormones, ACTH may be secreted by pituitary tumors and kidney tumors may produce erythropoietin.

More puzzling, is secretion of hormones by cancer cells which are derived from normal tissues which do not have this natural property. For example, some lung tumors produce ACTH and others have been incriminated in the secretion of antidiuretic hormone.[1] At times, characteristic symptoms produced are useful in diagnosing such conditions. However, since these symptoms are consistent with other non-neoplastic illnesses, care must be taken in forming a diagnosis.

The precise reasons underlying hormone production by otherwise non-endocrine tissues are not clear. Although all cells of the body have the same genotype, during normal differentiation, various portions of the genotype are suppressed. During early stages of cancer formation, de-repression of the genotype of some cells seems to occur. For example, some malignant cells are known to display embryonic antigens (Chap. 3), substances, otherwise elaborated during embryonic life and not thereafter. The synthesis of some hormones by tumors may be the result of the same phenomenon. For unknown reasons or as a result of unknown influences, repressed gene segments may be de-repressed, and transcription of DNA to protein can occur.

Whatever the mechanism, certain non-endocrine cancers have a greater tendency to hormone production than others, an element that further complicates this puzzling behavior. Again no reason is known, but an interesting pattern has been detected that perhaps sheds some light on this matter. Tumors originating from *less* differentiated cells, appear to have a greater propensity to synthesize hormones than neoplastic cells derived from highly specialized tissue. Conceivably, generalized tissues in which cells have a number of possible routes along which to differentiate have less rigid repression of their genotype when compared to those in which the routes of differentiation are more strictly circumscribed.

Toxic Substances. The metabolic byproducts of certain tumors seem to be toxic or at least pyrogenic. Fever is commonly associated with renal tumors and also with Hodgkin's disease. And, fever is caused by an intrinsic property of the disease itself, not by infectious complications,[2] although the precise mechanism by which it is mediated is unknown.[3,4]

Similarly unknown is the manner in which tumors produce neuropathy, usually of peripheral sensory nerves, or the manner by which thymic tumors become associated with myesthesia. However, in other cases, in which there are similar signs and symptoms, the mechanism is clear. For example, some tumors produce hypercalcemia, through either mechanical or chemical means, which in turn has a profound toxic effect on cerebral function.

Biochemical Abnormalities. Specific tumors may produce biochemical abnormalities, the reasons for which are not always clear and sometimes defy explanation.

Both hypo- and hyperglycemia have been reported with pancreatic cancers. Some insulin secreting pancreatic tumors produce hypoglycemia, but occasionally hepatomas,[5] adrenal cortical carcinomas, soft tissue sarcomas, gastric cancers and some lymphomas have been reported to produce the condition.

There is no certainty as to why hypoglycemia is caused by these cancers, but glucose consumption by the tumor may be responsible, liver function may be disturbed or tumors may cause changes in fat metabolism.

Another such phenomenon is the occurrence of thrombosis in persons with carcinoma.[6,7] Carcinomas of lung or pancreas seem especially prone to causing vascular thrombosis, particularly of vessels of the arm and neck. Precisely why this should be so is not known, although some authors believe that mucous-producing tumors increase coagulability and postulate this as a mechanism for the thrombi.

Another systemic reaction provoked by some tumors is elevation of erythrocyte sedimentation rate (E.S.R.). In particular, kidney and lung tumors, along with multiple myeloma can markedly elevate the E.S.R.

Still other biochemical changes are more specific. Some hepatomas and gonadal tumors produce an alpha-globulin called *Fetuin*. In a study of 38 patients with hepatoma, 68% had the fetoprotein, fetuin in blood sera.[8] The difference between persons with hepatoma who do or do not produce fetuin is not clear.

Still other tumors produce a variety of diverse and often unusual reactions. Some result in effects on complexion (pallor, jaundice), sensitivity to cold temperatures, changes in serum viscosity (pathological eyegrounds, venous dilation and engorgement, progressive vision impairment, nose and gum bleeds) and hemolysis of red cells. Others can cause flushing, diarrhea, borborygmus and/or wheezing. Still others release histamine leading to various degrees of hypersensitivity.

Nutritional Sequelae. A less specific type of change secondary to tumor is a general decrease in the nutritional status of the patient. Both tumor and effects secondary to anti-cancer therapy produce this change; however, in either case the result is the same. The patient becomes unable to maintain a positive nitrogen balance, as is necessary to deter tumor-induced damage, and, equally important, to support healing and compensate for tumor shrinkage during therapy.

The predominant manner in which a tumor affects nutritional status varies from cancer to cancer. Some anatomic sites are predisposed to specific problems. Lesions within the oral cavity frequently produce difficulty in chewing food or pain upon swallowing, inducing patients to decrease intake. Tumors of the hypopharynx and, in particular, the esophagus make swallowing difficult and at times impossible. Tumors of the lower gastrointestinal tract interfere with absorption of nutrients. Still other lesions produce effects through less obvious mechanisms. Advanced ovarian cancer characteristically gives rise to ascites, abdominal distention and cachexia. And, any type of tumor which has widely metastasized, especially to the liver, can produce anorexia. Last, one must not overlook the psychological effect of the diagnosis of cancer on the patient's appetite.

In addition, anti-cancer therapy often acts to interfere with adequate nutrition. Irradiation of the oral cavity can produce sufficient irritation to (1) make swallowing painful and difficult, (2) decrease salivary flow and (3) alter taste, all of which combine to decrease alimentary intake. If esophagus is within the treated field, esophagitis with its inherent symptom of a sensation of food "sticking" in the throat frequently occurs and the patient tends to limit intake. If the lower gastrointestinal tract is irritated, irritability, cramps, frequent stools and frank diarrhea may occur and decrease the patient's appetite.

Chemotherapeutic management can diminish nutrition. Methotrexate may produce significant irritation within the oral cavity making chewing or swallowing painful and difficult. 5-fluorouracil can induce diarrhea, and a large number of drugs frequently are associated with nausea and vomiting (as will be discussed in Chapter 16).

Part of cancer care, therefore, must deal with the maintenance of adequate nutrition. When the etiology of the problem is obvious, a specific answer may be sought. For example, when irradiation of the oral cavity is the problem, bland, room-temperature foods which are relatively well-tolerated, may be the solution (Table 16–4, p. 212). When mild dysphagia is present, soft, blenderized foods often can be tolerated when more conventional foods cannot. In other cases, where a particular problem/solution relationship does not exist, non-specific dietary changes can be tried. In general, the most substantial deficit is in protein balance, and easily swallowed, high protein supplements provide a partial answer. Simple mixtures, such as are obtained by dissolving powdered milk in regular milk, or only slightly more complicated milkshakes based upon milk, ice cream and eggs are examples of the kinds of nutritional supplements possible.[9] When dietary intake is sufficiently limited to preclude adequate nutrition despite supplemental feedings, alimentation via a nasogastric tube may be required. In still other situations, when absorption from the gastrointestinal tract is incompetent to support the patient's needs, intravenous feeding can be used to maintain nourishment.

Supportive Care. In light of the potentially devastating effects of both tumor and treatment, it should come as no surprise that afflicted patients need substantial supportive care. Discovering that you are a victim of cancer must be among the most terrifying events that can happen to a human being. It is the ultimate reminder of our mortality, for the average person has no ability to distinguish curable from incurable disease. Consequently, to a greater or lesser degree, all newly diagnosed patients require emotional support. They must be permitted to vent their anger and frustration in confronting, what may seem to them, an insoluble problem. They must be aided in arranging their affairs and preparing their families to take care of themselves during the period of testing and treatment and afterwards. At the same time, patients who are expected to recover from their illness must be encouraged to resume as many normal activities as possible. Outpatient chemotherapy and/or radiotherapy does not prevent most patients from returning to productive activities including work. To the extent that physical exercise is tolerated, it should be encouraged. The emotional boost of feeling useful, contributes immeasurably to the overall success of therapy.

A question that frequently arises is "how much should patients be told about their diagnosis?" Various opinions ranging from "almost nothing" to "almost everything" have been offered. However, in practice it is difficult to follow either policy for all patients.

We believe that patients have the fundamental right to be told as much about their diagnosis and prognosis as they can understand. It is vital to the doctor-patient relationship that a basic trust be established, and nothing short of absolute honesty between parties suffices to accomplish that end. On the other hand, there are many different ways of expressing an idea, and it is in this context that the medical staff has the greatest number of options and, therefore, the largest potential to create a positive therapeutic environment. A professional demeanor and a positive attitude can be powerful weapons. In the process of explaining the ramifications of disease and treatment to the patient, hope should not be crushed. The potential benefits of treatment should be stressed and the patient must be given sufficient encouragement to have the will to resist being disabled.

Every patient must be allowed to indicate precisely how much detail he wishes to know and can comprehend. It is not necessary (and certainly not beneficial) to inflict all details of adverse responses to and outcomes of treatments at first meeting. The patient who tells you he knows he has "a tumor" need not be reminded in callous detail that he has a potentially lethal cancer. Nothing good will be accomplished and, at times, unnecessarily bleak expectations will be aroused. This philosophy applies even to the patient who is incurable and is receiving treatment solely for palliation. Far more is gained by telling such patients that measures can be taken to make them comfortable, than by telling them they have but a short time left to live. The patient who asks a direct question should receive a direct answer, even if it is unpleasant, but sufficient time should be allowed for patients to adjust to the shock of reality and to assimilate details of their illness at a rate which permits them to cope.

The above comments by no means apply solely to physicians. Every member of the oncology team must bear the same responsibility. In fact, the frequently closer rapport between patient and nurse than between patient and doctor compels the nursing staff to accept much of the responsibility for such work. Reinforcement of these concepts by all who come into contact with the patient is essential. In part, the attitude must be generated even from inanimate objects. The patient takes keys from all parts of his environment, and it is not uncommon to have patients relate that their only recollection of receiving radiation therapy is of lying on a cold table, *all alone*, in a deadly quiet room. Chemotherapy patients can so associate side effects of treatment with their surroundings, that some become nauseated just by walking into the office or clinic. To ameliorate some of this, care must be taken even in the manner in which the facility is decorated. Colors should be bright and cheerful and, at the same time, soothing and warm. Symbols of life, such as plants or tropical fish, should be liberally distributed throughout. Paintings should reflect pleasant subject matter and avoid somber colors, still lifes and abstracts that might be interpreted as a disfigured person. Softly played, gentle music also can create a positive environment.

To complement this psychological support, substantial physical care is required. Cancer victims require the routine nursing care commonly afforded patients having other diagnoses and, at times, demand intensive attention. Most specifically, tumors and their treatment create unique problems requiring specialized oncologic nursing care before, during and after therapy.

Prior to treatment, patients must be prepared properly for what is to come. Few know what to expect and how best to cope. For example, patients who are about to undergo radiotherapy should know that they will not feel anything during treatment. Patients who are going to be taking cyclophosphamide must be advised to insure an abundant intake of fluids to dilute the toxic effects of the drug on the urinary bladder. When treatment begins, as a preventative measure, patients must be instructed in methods of proper skin care of areas being irradiated and must be helped in taking care of reactions that may arise from either radiotherapy or chemotherapy (Chap. 16). Perhaps most important, because of the lack of general appreciation of the need for subsequent care, patients must be indoctrinated with the concept. For example, women who receive irradiation of the vagina as part of treatment for vaginal, cervical or endometrial carcinoma, are prone to develop adhesions and contraction of the vagina because of radiation induced changes. To ameliorate such reactions, the proper use of lubricated vaginal dilators and well-defined programs of vaginal hygiene should be taught and enforced. In short, oncologic care must be directed to the entire person, not just the tumor.

References

1. Klein, L.A., Rabson, A.S. and Worksman, J.: In Vitro Synthesis of Vasopressin by Lung Tumor Cells. Surgical Forum *20*:231–233, 1969.
2. Lobell, M., Boggs, D.R. and Wintrobe, M.M.: The Clinical Significance of Fever in Hodgkin's Disease. Arch. Intern. Med. *117*:335–342, 1966.
3. Rawlins, M.D., Luff, R.H. and Crauston, W.I.: Pyrexia in Renal Carcinoma. Lancet *1*:1371–1373, 1970.
4. Bodel, P.: Tumors and Fever. In Hall, T. (Ed): Paraneoplastic Syndromes: Ann. N. Y. Acad. Sci. *230*:6–13, 1974.
5. McFadzean, A.J.S. and Yeung, R.T.T.: Further Observations on Hypoglycemia and Hepatocellular Carcinoma. Am. J. Med. *47*:220–235, 1969.
6. Fisher, M.M., Hockberg, L.A. and Wilensky, N.D.: Recurrent Thrombophlebitis in Obscure Malignant Tumor of the Lung. J.A.M.A. *147*:1213–1216, 1951.
7. Lieberman, J.S., Barrero, J. and Vidarreta, E.: Thrombophlebitis and Cancer. J.A.M.A. *177*:542–545, 1961.
8. Waldenstrom, J.F.: *Pareneoplasia. Biological Signals in the Diagnosis of Cancer.* New York, John Wiley & Sons, 1978, p. 76.
9. Nutrition for Patients Receiving Chemotherapy and Radiation Treatment. New York, The American Cancer Society, 1974.

THE
HAZARDS

16

ACUTE REACTIONS

From previous discussions, it should be clear that differences between neoplastic and normal cells are small and that any attempt to kill neoplastic cells is likely to damage if not kill normal cells, too. Damage to normal cells is frequently evident during and shortly after treatment and expresses itself as a *reaction*. In general, these changes are basically annoying, usually transient and do not risk the life of the patient.

The purpose of this chapter is to discuss the more common reactions to therapy. We have included only those reactions the non-specialist is likely to see and have suggested commonly accepted management.

General Comments. Nausea, vomiting, anorexia and lethargy are the symptoms most commonly associated with anti-cancer therapy. However, the degree to which any of these symptoms is present, depends on location and size of field irradiated or chemotherapeutic agent used, the dose of either and individual tolerance of the patient. Many chemotherapeutic agents are common offenders and produce all four symptoms (Table 16–1). By contrast, nausea and vomiting are

Table 16–1. Chemotherapeutic Agents Which Commonly Induce Nausea

Actinomycin	Melphalan
Adriamycin	Mithromycin
Bleomycin	Mitomycin-C
Chlorambucil	Nitrogen Mustard
Cyclophosphamide	Nitrosoureas (BCNU, CCNU, Me-CCNU)
Cis-platinum	Procarbazine
Hexamethylmelamine	Streptozotocin
Imidazole Carboxamide	Thiotepa

unusual side effects of radiotherapy except when the upper abdomen is being treated. At times, lethargy is related to prolonged nausea and vomiting; however, patients receiving either radiotherapy or chemotherapy not infrequently complain of decreased energy even when they do not feel ill. Yet, with the exception of patients who require hospitalization because of their disease and those patients on aggressive multidrug programs requiring intensive supportive care, most patients can be treated as outpatients, and many manage to return to work during therapy. Treatment of these symptoms basically is palliative; reassurance, antiemetic medication, rest as needed and, occasionally, moderation of dose.

Fever is an unusual side effect of treatment. When it occurs shortly after administration of parenteral chemotherapy, contamination of the drug should be considered. However, some drugs in and of themselves occasionally produce fever. Daunorubicin (daunomycin) can do this, L-asparaginase may produce an allergic response characterized by fever, chills and urticaria and imidazole carboxamide (DTIC) can produce an infectious-looking picture of fever, malaise and myalgia.

External beam radiotherapy rarely produces fever although, at least in theory, rapid necrosis of a tumor could lead to liberation of sufficient pyrogens to induce fever. On the other hand, intracavitary irradiation of cervical carcinoma frequently is associated with low grade fever. While it responds to antipyretics, this may mask a more catastrophic event, such as perforation of the uterus, and prophylactic or routine treatment is not recommended. In contrast, when fever is secondary to the neoplasm itself, as occurs in Hodgkin's disease, appropriate anti-cancer therapy can bring about defevesence.

In view of concern frequently expressed by patients, we mention here one reaction which does *not* occur. Patients receiving external beam radiotherapy do *not* become radioactive and present no danger to their families or friends. Patients treated by insertion or implantation of radioactive materials transmit some radiation through their bodies and consequently are routinely confined to hospital in private rooms, isolated from other patients. When permanent implants are used, isotopes with short half lives in small amounts are placed in their bodies. The isotopes decay and virtually are not radioactive when such persons are allowed to leave the hospital. They present no danger to the public

Skin. Cells of normal epithelium constantly undergo a maturational process characterized by movement from the deepest, basal layer to the most superficial, keratin layer, and as they move, change in morphology and function. Every 4 weeks, the keratin layer is shed and replaced by cells originating in the basal layer. If basal cells are damaged or destroyed and shedding of keratin continues, orderly replacement may not be possible.

External beam radiotherapy always passes through some portion of the skin to reach the tumor, thus damaging skin. In fact, in the past, clinical manifestations of this damage were used as the standard of dose in radiotherapy. Today this effect is ameliorated by the skin sparing of megavoltage equipment and the use of moving beam and multiportal therapy, but some skin damage still exists. Proper skin care can avoid clinical problems. Table 16–2 is a copy of some of the instructions given patients receiving irradiation at New York University Medical Center.

Clinically, the most common skin reaction to radiation is *erythema* secondary to dermal capillary congestion. While this reaction can be seen after as little as one treatment; in general, assuming common dose/time/fractionation schemes it is clinically evident usually after 2 to 3 weeks of daily treatment. The reaction is generally asymptomatic and requires no treatment. Occasionally, patients experience itching within the treatment field which can be moderated by application of a thin coating of corn starch.

If treatment continues, damaged and dead cells begin to accumulate. At this point the skin appears dry, and if it is gently brushed, will *desquamate* flakes of skin. In addition, irradiation stimulates enzymatic production of melanin giving the skin a dark appearance, par-

Table 16–2. Care of Skin During and After Radiation Therapy

---

1. SKIN MARKS ARE NECESSARY FOR THE ACCURATE POSITIONING OF TREATMENT AND MUST NOT BE WASHED OFF. However,
2. Gentle daily washing of the treatment area is permitted using WARM *WATER ONLY*. Pat dry—DO NOT RUB. If reaction occurs from radiation and the treated area becomes red and itchy, it should be kept DRY and lightly dusted with CORN STARCH.
3. NO creams, soaps, ointments, lotions or deodorants should be applied to the treated area without permission.
4. Avoid any tight clothing such as collars, girdles or belts which may cause friction in the treated area. Do not wear wool next to the skin in the treated area.
5. Heating pads or ice packs should NOT be used in the treated area.
6. AVOID direct, constant sunshine on the area during treatment. NO SUNBATHING without permission. Ask the physician about long-term skin care.

---

ticularly around each hair follicle.[1] Most patients are asymptomatic and require no treatment at this point.

Sometimes clinical circumstances dictate continued therapy in the face of this dry desquamation. If sufficient damage within the basal cell layer is incurred, the keratin layer will not be replaced and the integrity of the epithelial barrier will be lost. As a result part or all of the irradiated area will become moist from leakage of serum. This reaction, moist desquamation, should prompt a change in radiotherapeutic technique to decrease damage to the basal cell layer. In time, if no further damge occurs, the area will epithelialize from its periphery and cells of hair follicles will appear (which are relatively resistant to damage) within the irradiated portal. In addition, application of a soothing protective barrier such as hydrophilic petrolatum (aquaphor) and telpha coated dressings promote healing. Occasionally, topical steroids or antiseptics can be of value, but their use should be at the discretion of the responsible radiation oncologist.

Dermatologic reactions secondary to chemotherapy do not occur frequently; however, they can happen. Bleomycin is the most likely etiologic agent, sometimes resulting in desquamation of the hands, feet and other areas subject to stress, with occasional bullae formation, hyperpigmentation, pruritic erythema and ridging of the nails. Hyperpigmentation appears to be a "standard" response to several agents including busulfan, cyclophosphamide, 5-fluorouracil, actinomycin-D, and procarbazine. Unusual reactions are ridged nails (cyclophosphamide), maculopapular rashes (hydroxyurea) and acneform eruptions (actinomycin-D, steroids). Unquestionably, the most striking reaction occurs from the synergistic actions of some drugs with radiation. Actinomycin-D is a prime example. In combination with radiation it results in strikingly more intense, more frequent radiation-type reactions than would be expected from radiation alone. Moreover, the drug and radiation need not be given concomitantly. Actinomycin-D, given long after the acute reaction to irradiation has subsided, will "recall" these reactions within the treated region. Conversely, a patient who has received actinomycin-D in the past must be irradiated cautiously.

Hair. Hair follicles also are frequently affected by treatment. The most obvious change secondary to radiotherapy is epilatioh. The kelihbood of this change is dependent upon the anatomic site irradiated nd appears to correlate with rate of hair growth at that site. acas agne and G icouroff[2] noted progressively decreasing sensitivity to epilation in the following order: scalp, male beard, eyebrows, axilla, pubis, and the fine hairs over the body. It usually takes 2 to 3 weeks after the initiation of radiotherapy for epilation to become noticeable. If the total dose is relatively low (as in prophylactic treatment of acute lymphocytic leukemia), regrowth characteristically occurs within 4 to 6 months after treatment; however, if the total dose is relatively high (as in treatment of a primary glioma), epilation may be permanent. In addition, irradiation may change the color of hair, whether or not epilation occurs.

Alopecia secondary to chemotherapy is common with several drugs, namely cyclophosphamide, actinomycin-D, adriamycin and daunomycin. Drugs which less frequently cause this change are methotrexate, 5-fluorouracil, vinblastine, vincristine, mitomycin-C, CCNU, methyl-CCNU, imidazole carboxamide, and hydroxyurea. Some authors have advocated using a scalp tourniquet during administration of drugs to prevent alopecia.

Oral Mucosa. Because mucosa of the oral cavity is similar to skin in terms of structure and function, it is perhaps not surprising that when irradiated, its behavior is similar to that of skin. In contrast to skin, however, cells of the mucosal epithelium have a shorter life span, and therefore more rapid maturation. Consequently equivalent amounts of damage to the skin and mucosa will produce a clinical reaction in the mucosa sooner. On the other hand, reactions in the oral cavity heal more rapidly than those of skin. Because of the rapidity with which reactions can occur, and the marked pain they bring, it is extremely important to urge patients to give up tobacco and alcohol during treatment. The continued use of these irritants substantially increases severity and frequency of these reactions and can be the difference between successful completion of therapy as planned and the need to suspend or modify treatment. Tables 16–3 and 4 are a copy of some of the instructions given to patients who are treated to the head and neck area.

Early in treatment there usually is no reaction in the mouth or only slight erythema. As treatment continues, the degree of erythema increases and after a few weeks small patches of grey-white mucositis may form. This can progress until the patches coalesce forming large painful patches not suited to serve as a barrier to irritants and pathogens. Treatment of such lesions requires a change in radiotherapeutic technique and symptomatic relief. A wide variety of palliatives work and the efficacy of each and, indeed, the treatment of choice depends

Table 16–3.   Daily Care for Patients Undergoing Treatment to the Head and Neck

1. SKIN MARKS ARE NECESSARY FOR THE ACCURATE POSITIONING OF TREATMENT AND MUST NOT BE WASHED OFF. However,
2. Gentle daily washing of the treatment area is permitted using WARM *WATER ONLY*. Pat dry—DO NOT RUB. If reaction occurs from radiation and the treated area becomes red and itchy, it should be kept DRY and lightly dusted with CORN STARCH.
3. SMOKING IS *NOT* PERMITTED if the mouth or throat is being treated.
4. It is generally wise to avoid alcohol, but beer, wine and well-diluted spirits may be allowed—ask permission.
5. You may shave GENTLY in the treated area using an ELECTRIC RAZOR ONLY. Do not use pre- or after shave lotions.
6. Makeup should not be used in the treated area.
7. If the scalp is being treated, ask for instructions about washing the hair.
8. AVOID spicy or seasoned foods, or scratchy foods such as bacon, celery, toast, etc. which may irritate the throat. A semi-soft diet with supplemental feedings (Table 16–4) should be followed if swallowing becomes difficult.
9. Instead of mouth wash, gargle one teaspoonful of baking soda in ½ glass of WARM water 3 or 4 times a day.

Table 16–4.   Sample Semi-Soft Diet

BREAKFAST
    4 ounces pear nectar, 1 cup cooked farina, 1 scrambled egg, 1 slice buttered toast, jelly, 1 cup fortified milk, coffee, ½ ounce cream, 2 teaspoons sugar.

LUNCH
    Creamed soup, 2 ounces ground roast beef, gravy, ½ cup mashed potatoes, ½ cup buttered carrots, 1 slice buttered bread, chocolate pudding, 1 cup fortified milk, coffee, ½ ounce cream, 2 teaspoons sugar.

DINNER
    2 ounces ground chicken, ½ cup buttered noodles, ½ cup green peas, 1 slice buttered bread, ½ cup applesauce, 1 cup fortified milk, coffee, ½ ounce cream, 2 teaspoons sugar.

SUPPLEMENTAL FEEDINGS

FORTIFIED MILK—1 cup milk, ⅓ cup instant nonfat dry milk, mix well

HIGH PROTEIN EGGNOG—1 cup milk, 2 eggs, ⅓ cup nonfat dry milk, 1 teaspoon vanilla. Beat egg well, add part of milk and dry milk. Dissolve, add rest of milk, vanilla and sugar to taste.

HIGH PROTEIN MILKSHAKE—1 cup milk, 1 scoop ice cream, ⅓ cup instant nonfat dry milk (for malt add 2 teaspoons malt). Flavor: 2 tablespoons chocolate syrup, 1 teaspoon vanilla or 2 tablespoons coffee. Dissolve dry milk in milk, add flavoring and ice cream. Beat well.

on the individual patient. Soft, non-spiced foods served at room temperature, coatings such as olive oil, topical analgesics and a prescribed program of oral hygiene to decrease the chance of superinfection, are all helpful.

Stomatitis can be caused by chemotherapeutic drugs, in particular, methotrexate. In fact, oral stomatitis is often the first sign of methotrexate toxicity and the dose limiting factor in such treatment. Other drugs which may produce moderate to severe stomatitis are 5-fluorouracil, actinomycin-D, adriamycin, cytosine arabinoside, vinblastine, mitomycin-C, CCNU, imidazole carboxamide and procarbazine. Again, treatment consists of withdrawal or at least moderation of the offending agent and symptomatic relief.

Salivary Glands and Taste. When the oral cavity is treated by external beam radiotherapy, the parotid glands frequently are irradiated too. This results in a marked reduction of serous output. Saliva becomes thick, tenacious and oral pH changes. It is surprising how much this distresses the patient. Some relief is afforded by mouthwashes which thin and dissolve these secretions. A simple but effective mouthwash can be made from 1 teaspoon of bicarbonate of soda dissolved in ½ glass of warm water.

In addition to changing the quality of saliva, irradiation decreases acuity of the taste buds. In particular, the ability to taste sweet is diminished, and patients often alter their diets to include more carbohydrates. In combination with salivary changes, the high carbohydrate diet increases the risk of subsequent dental decay as will be discussed in the next chapter.

Nervous Tissue. The brain and spinal cord usually exhibit no acute reaction to treatment. Although the possibility that irradiation of tissue could induce edema formation which if trapped within a closed space (the cranial bones) could lead to increased (intracranial) pressure, if this occurs at a clinically detectable level at all, it must be uncommon. Rubin[3] measured spinal fluid pressure before and after irradiation and could find no evidence of "radiation induced edema." Perhaps whatever edema does form is a residue of destroyed neoplastic cells and occupies the space that such cells leave.

Patients who receive irradiation for primary brain tumors do have to be monitored for reaction, but not in the brain itself. Approximately 10% of such patients experience radiation induced otitis media which responds to conventional treatment. In addition, the cutaneous reaction behind the ears can be intense because of the lessening of the skin sparing effect of high energy irradiation due to the ear itself. Bending the ear forward on alternate days during radiation decreases this problem.

Two late reactions merit discussion. One is a syndrome associated with low dose cranial irradiation for prophylaxis against leukemia in children. Approximately 6 weeks after such treatment, children can experience a 1 week interval of lethargy, somnolence and low grade fever which requires no treatment and clears spontaneously. The other is a syndrome characterized by electric-like sensations in the hands and/or feet occurring several months after irradiation of the spinal cord. Symptoms may be elicited by flexion of the head, and patients may comment (only incidentally) that they experience an unusual sensation when they look down at the curb before crossing a street. The prognostic importance of this reaction, commonly called *L'hermittes syndrome*, is uncertain. Although some patients proceed to develop spinal cord complications, in most cases, the syndrome is self-limiting and no further problems develop.

In general, systemic chemotherapy does not penetrate the blood-brain barrier and no acute reactions would be expected or are seen. Occasionally procarbazine produces lethargy and drowsiness. More rarely there is hyperexcitability—up to and including convulsions—or peripheral neuropathy. Other drugs which may lead to nervous system reactions are L-asparaginase which can produce lethargy, somno-lence, impaired mentation and, rarely, coma, and 5-fluorouracil which occasionally produces cerebellar ataxia. When chemotherapy is delivered by the intrathecal route, sterile meningitis can result. Methotrexate, as used for acute leukemia, not uncommonly produces transient headache and backache, with or without nausea and vomit-ing. The most specific acute reactions to treatment are displayed by peripheral and cranial nerves to the administration of vincristine and cis-platinum. Patients who receive vincristine often complain of "pins and needles" in their fingertips. Almost invariably, an early sign of toxicity is the loss of the "ankle-jerk" deep tendon reflex. Intestinal motility can also be neurologically compromised. Cis-platinum on the other hand is toxic to the eighth cranial nerve resulting in hearing loss. Appropriate treatment of these neuropathies is withdrawal or modera-tion of the drug.

Blood and Bone Marrow. The acute toxicity of most chemo-therapeutic agents is seen in the reaction of the hematologic system.

Table 16–5.   Chemotherapeutic Drugs Which Have Substantial Marrow Toxicity

actinomycin-D	melphalan
adriamycin	6-mercaptopurine
BCNU	methotrexate
busulfan	methyl CCNU
CCNU	mithramycin
chlorambucil	mitomycin-C
cis-platinum	nitrogen mustard
cyclophosphamide	procarbazine
daunomycin	6-thioguanine
5-fluorouracil	thiotepa
hydroxyurea	vinblastine

Leukopenia and/or thrombocytopenia are so frequent with many drugs (Table 16–5) that their *absence* raises the suspicion that the patient is being undertreated. *Mild* cytopenias are no more an indication to withhold chemotherapy than is a mild skin reaction an indication to withhold radiotherapy. Of course, moderate decreases in blood count dictate need for reduced doses and marked cytopenia requires suspension of therapy.

The nitrosoureas deserve individual consideration because of the pattern of marrow toxicity they induce. Unlike other drugs which cause a relatively rapid decrease, the height of the reaction to nitrosoureas occurs 4 to 6 weeks after treatment. Failure to appreciate this pattern can lead to inappropriate administration of drugs just before the nadir in blood count in the belief that adequate marrow support exists.

Perhaps surprisingly, most radiotherapeutic regimens do *not* induce clinical cytopenia. Although some circulating cells must be destroyed, rarely must therapy be altered to suit marrow tolerance. There are some notable exceptions to this general rule. Large fields which include large percentages of the functioning marrow such as are necessary for total nodal irradiation in Hodgkin's disease, entire abdomen irradiation of ovarian carcinoma, half-body irradiation for palliation of painful diffuse metastases or whole body irradiation for active leukemia require attention to blood count.

Although some ultra-aggressive multi-drug protocols may require support of hematologic reactions by transfusion of specific blood fractions, the type of treatment programs which involve the non-oncologist, should not require any treatment other than suspension or moderation of the offending therapy.

Lung. Depending upon volume of lung irradiated and dose achieved, pulmonary reactions to radiation therapy may occur. After a few weeks, inflammatory changes (congestion, exudation and infiltration by white blood cells) begin, peaking at 1 month post treatment. Frequently, such patients are asymptomatic, although some develop cough and slight fever, possibly secondary to associated infection. Treatment requires symptomatic care, evaluation for associated infection and, depending on results, treatment of associated infection.

Esophagus. The epithelial lining of the esophagus reacts to irradiation by inflammatory response which sometimes produces dysphagia. At 2 to 3 weeks into treatment, dysphagia becomes evident but fortunately resolves spontaneously in 7 to 10 days, despite continued irradiation. During the symptomatic phase, topical analgesia may be helpful. Having the patient swallow one-half glassful of warm water which contains two dissolved aspirins is usually effective.

Abdomen and Pelvis. As previously mentioned, irradiation of the upper abdomen can produce nausea, vomiting and anorexia. It is important to maintain adequate nutrition despite these symptoms, and a high protein, bland diet should be prescribed. Antiemetics may prove necessary. When this region is treated, the radiation oncologist may have to titrate the daily dose against the patient's symptoms, just as the medical oncologist titrates daily drug dose by blood count. When the lower abdomen is treated, cramps with or without an increased number of bowel movements per day can result. At New York University Medical Center, all such patients are prophylactically placed on a low residue diet (Table 16–6) during therapy. In addition, if the patient becomes symptomatic, antispasmodic medications, antidiarrheal medications and dose modifications are used when appropriate. Diarrhea secondary to chemotherapy is most frequent with 5-fluorouracil, methotrexate and actinomycin-D but can occur to a milder degree with 6-mercaptopurine, vinblastine, adriamycin, imidazole carboxamide and procarbazine.

Bladder. Irradiation of the bladder can create sufficient irritation to result in urinary frequency, urgency and burning on urination. Soothing agents such as pyridium are helpful; however, it is imperative to rule out a superimposed bacterial infection. Should infection be present, appropriate antibiotics are mandatory. Cystitis secondary to cy-

Table 16–6.   Restricted Residue Diet

This diet avoids mechanical irritation of the gastrointestinal tract by restricting foods containing indigestible carbohydrate and tough connective tissue. It is adequate in all nutrients, provides foods which are non-irritating, easily digested and leaves a minimum of residue in the intestine.

FOOD GROUPS	FOODS ALLOWED	FOODS TO AVOID
Beverages	Milk (no more than 3 cups daily), coffee, tea, cocoa, decaffeinated coffee, carbonated beverages.	All others.
Bread	White, crackers, melba toast (all without seeds).	Bread containing bran or coarse whole grain; rolls, pancakes, waffles, quick breads.
Cereals	Refined cooked cereals (cream of rice, cream of wheat, farina, grits, strained oatmeal). Dry cereals (corn flakes, puffed rice, rice krispies, sugar smacks, special K).	All others.
Desserts	Angel food or sponge cake; plain cakes with simple icing, plain cookies, ice cream, sherbet, fruit whips, gelatine, puddings (bread, cornstarch, rice, tapioca), custard.	Rich pastries, cakes and puddings; desserts containing nuts, coconut or any fruits.
Eggs	Any way except fried.	Fried eggs.
Fats	Butter, margarine, cream.	All others.
Soups	Broth, consomme, creamed soups made with pureed vegetables.	All others.
Cheese	Cottage, cream cheese, mild American cheese.	All others.

clophosphamide can be severe and patients receiving this drug must be cautioned to maintain adequate fluid intake.

References

1. Moss. W.T., Brand, W.N. and Battifora, H.: *Radiation Oncology–Rationale, Technique, Results.* St. Louis, The C. V. Mosby Co., 1973, p. 86.
2. Ibid, p. 58.
3. Rubin, P.: Extradural Spinal Cord Compression by Tumor. Radiology 93:1243–1248, 1969.

17
COMPLICATIONS

Complications result when permanent damage to normal tissue, acquired during therapy, becomes clinically evident. Damage can affect any organ system and depending upon the site involved, produces a wide range of disabilities, including reparable ones (such as cataract formation) and irreparable ones (such as spinal cord necrosis), but only those organs that absorb damage in excess of their capacity to repair will manifest these changes. By now tolerance to damage of various organs is reasonably well established; unfortunately, tolerance often occurs at or near dose levels required for control of disease. Thus, treatment usually involves an element of risk; one must hope that the patient's normal tissues are not unexpectedly sensitive or the tumor tissue unexpectedly insensitive, since either may result in an undesirable outcome.

But, for the moment, consider the worst possible outcome of therapy. What is it? What type of complication is intolerable? Isn't it failure to cure the potentially curable patient? Ironically, juries routinely tend to award substantial sums to patients who are cured of disease, but injured by therapy, while settlement for failure to cure disease would be a rarity. Yet, risk of complications could virtually be eliminated by decreasing intensity of treatment and allowing more victims to die. While this hypothetical stratagem is both unconscionable and unacceptable, it is purposely stated to force consideration of the alternatives. Surely, there are methods of complication prevention and a high rate of complications is to be condemned, *but* a low incidence of complications must be seen as an unavoidable byproduct of *appropriate* therapy.

In addition, the concept of "a complication" is not absolute and application of the word sometimes can be misleading. For example, a child who is cured of retinoblastoma by surgical enucleation becomes "blind" in that eye—as an accepted part of treatment. In contrast, a similar child who is cured by irradiation, but develops a cataract obscuring vision in that eye, is commonly stated to have had a complication of treatment. Thus, what constitutes an integral part of treatment versus a complication of treatment at times can be debated.

However, complications do occur and when they do, present a substantial problem to the patient and to everyone involved in his or her care. The purpose of this chapter is to describe the more common complications of treatment by non-surgical oncologic methods. It is our hope that by describing them, the likelihood of their occurrence, their usual severity and their appropriate management, we can help the reader minimize their effect.

Complications vs. Cure. The likelihood of complications for the average patient varies as a function of dose (and for radiotherapy, the volume irradiated). Usually the incidence follows a relation similar to that already described for sterilization of disease. At lower doses, complications are few and the incidence of complications does not rise dramatically with small increments in dose. However, at some point, tissue tolerance is reached and the incidence of complications rises rapidly. Eventually, so many patients have complications that additional therapy produces only a small change. At any dose level, however, there always will be some chance of complications.

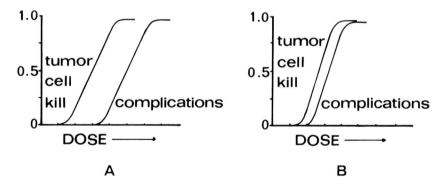

Fig. 17–1.   *Relationship of tumor cell kill and production of complications to dose in two hypothetical situations. A. Tumor cells are killed by lower doses than produce complications. In other words, a dose can be selected at which a high likelihood of tumor sterilization can be achieved with few complications. B. Complications tend to occur almost as frequently as does tumor cell sterilization at any given dose. A dose cannot be selected that is likely to cure disease without inducing complications.*

The efficacy of therapy depends largely on the ability to kill tumor cells without inducing complications at any given dose. When the cure curve is distant from the complication curve, as in Figure 17–1A, a dose can be chosen which will yield a high likelihood of cure with a low percentage of complications. However, when the curves closely approximate, as in Figure 17–1B, the same chance of cure entails a much higher risk of complications, or conversely, the same risk of complications will produce few cures. Whether optimal treatment for a hypothetical situation would be acceptance of a 70% cure rate with a 5% complication rate, an 80% cure rate with a 25% complication rate or a 95% cure rate with a 75% complication rate is an unsettled point. However, it is probably fair to assume that prior to treatment most patients would happily trade the acceptance of a complication for a guarantee of cure.

The Complications. Complications can occur in any part of the body but tend to occur at certain sites more frequently than would be expected by chance. What accounts for this distribution is the wide variation in sensitivity to damage of various organs. Because the oncologist must respect tolerance of the most sensitive structures affected by treatment, other less sensitive organs rarely sustain clinically apparent damage. Thus, the non-oncologist is likely to see complications only in the more sensitive organs, from head to toe, as follows.

Central Nervous System. Complications arising in the central nervous system rarely occur. In part this is explained by the ability of neural tissue to resist damage. In addition, when complications do occur, they are so severe in nature that the oncologist takes great pains to keep their incidence at an absolute minimum. For example, during the 36-year period from 1931 to 1967 only 57 cases of radiation induced brain necrosis were reported in the medical literature, and of these, 19 were secondary to treatment of extracranial tumors and an additional 10 developed only after repeated courses of high dose irradiation.[1]

Kramer and Lee[2] have reviewed the subject of radiation induced CNS complications. Although there is some debate about the pathophysiology, the primary change appears to be a disruption of fine vasculature of the brain and/or spinal cord. Several factors implicate this mechanism. *First*, brain or cord necrosis usually manifests itself 6 months to 3 years after irradiation (direct neural damage probably would be evident sooner). *Second*, radiation induced necrosis primarily affects cerebral white matter and the upper thoracic spinal cord, presumably due to limitations of their blood supply. *Last*, when necrosis occurs, small vessel damage is a consistent histopathologic finding.

Clinically, radiation induced brain damage has no pathognomonic signs or symptoms. Cerebral necrosis can be manifest in the same fashion as a recurrent tumor or a localized infection. Radiographic studies frequently demonstrate a "mass," but rarely differentiate between tumor, infection or necrosis. Sometimes, angiography will demonstrate vascular occlusion, suggesting the correct etiology, but, in general, cerebral necrosis is a diagnosis of exclusion. Finding necrosis on biopsy is not conclusive, as anaplastic brain tumors characteristically exhibit such areas, even in the absence of any therapy.

Radiation necrosis of spinal cord can be diagnosed with greater assurance. Clinically, it presents as motor and sensory deficits, which point to the affected anatomic level which must correspond to the site of irradiation. Although epidural tumor, or a paraneoplastic syndrome need be considered, the occurrence of a lesion at the site of high dose irradiation, 6 months to 3 years after treatment, suggests radiation necrosis. In addition, a normal myelogram virtually rules out epidural metastases.

The Eye. The eyes are complex structures, composed of several different types of tissue. Most of the eye resists radiation induced damage; however, the lens is one of the most radiosensitive structures in the body. At low doses, considerably below the minimum dose required for sterilization of any malignant tumor, cataract formation which may or may not progress to produce visual impairment frequently occurs.[3] Cells at the equator of the lens are damaged and, when, in the normal course of events they migrate posteriorly, produce opacities in the otherwise clear lens. In fact, the cataract's characteristics are unique and an ophthalmologist visually can distinguish a radiation-induced cataract from the more common cataract associated with aging.

At high dose levels, other structures can incur damage, leading to retinal degeneration, optic nerve atrophy, central artery thrombosis and blindness, although such changes rarely are seen. Shukovsky and Fletcher[1] noted these complications only after aggressive irradiation of adjacent structures, such as sometimes is required in the treatment of maxillary sinus cancer.

Radiation induced cataracts can be removed by the same procedures used for spontaneous cataracts. More extensive damage may be temporized but usually cannot be repaired.

Oral Cavity. Complications within the oral cavity can involve many different structures including mucous membranes, bones, salivary glands, teeth and taste buds. The pathophysiology of damage to each site differs as do the complications and their therapy.

Mucous membranes of the mouth resist radiation or chemotherapy induced damage relatively well as was discussed in Chapter 16. However, when tolerance is exceeded, ulceration can occur. In most cases, conservative management will suffice. Oral hygiene measures must be enforced by means of topical dilute hydrogen peroxide mouth washes, pressure sprays, antibiotics and analgesics. Most cases, particularly if bone is not involved and the ulcer is not large, will heal with this regimen, rarely requiring surgical therapy.

Damage to bone has become less common as a result of improved radiotherapeutic equipment. While producing the same dose within an intra-oral tumor, current megavoltage equipment delivers a lower dose to bone than did previous kilovoltage equipment. Another factor which significantly influences incidence of bone complications is the status of bone prior to treatment; if tumor has invaded bone, the chance of osteonecrosis is greater, the management more difficult and prognosis worse than osteonecrosis in a bone uninvolved by tumor. Rubin and Casarett[5] suggest the terms "complicated osteoradionecrosis" for the former situation as opposed to "simple osteoradionecrosis" for the latter. In addition, these authors provide an excellent detailed discussion for the reader who requires additional information.

Clinically, osteoradionecrosis develops fairly rapidly after treatment. MacComb[6] found that three-quarters of all cases of osteonecrosis occurred within the first year after treatment. Patients complain of severe pain and a tender irregular ulcer crater develops. Radiographically, mandibular necrosis is difficult to distinguish from recurrent disease. Sclerosis, mottled areas of resorption or osteoporosis may represent either recurrent disease or osteoradionecrosis.

Treatment of osteonecrosis, when recurrent or persistent tumor is *not* present, is similar to treatment of mucous membrane ulceration. Pressure sprays and irrigation with mild mouth washes, should be used to effect hygiene. If necessary, the spread of necrosis can be tempered and healing promoted by application of a paste composed of a topical antibiotic and a mild corticosteroid, mixed in a carrier such as carboxymethylcellulose. Conservative measures should be tried first in every patient with osteoradionecrosis. Surgical intervention should not be attempted unless a proper persistent trial of conservative measures has proved ineffective.

In addition, measures should be taken subsequent to therapy to minimize the risk of osteonecrosis. A retrospective analysis of the patients at the M. D. Anderson Hospital[7] revealed that 60% of cases of osteonecrosis had a precipitating cause such as dental extractions, mandibular surgery or an irritating prosthesis in the irradiated area, all of which should be avoided whenever possible.

Damage to the teeth as a result of irradiation, results less from direct damage than from secondary changes. After 1 week of irradiation, average salivary flow rates decrease approximately 50%, after 6 weeks, almost 75%—and may remain decreased for years after treatment.[8] At the same time, irradiation decreases acuity of taste buds and patients frequently alter their diets to include more carbohydrates and sweets. Last, either because of pain from the lesion itself, discomfort from treatment, or both, patients are reticent to employ vigorous oral hygiene measures during treatment. All these changes contribute to a change in saliva (which becomes more acidic) and lead to increased risk of dental decay and subsequent osteonecrosis. Once these changes have occurred, restorative dentistry becomes extremely difficult. Consequently, prophylactic measures to prevent such changes are becoming established as standard routines in many radiotherapy centers. Prior to treatment all patients should have dental evaluation. Teeth should be thoroughly cleaned and simple restorative dentistry done. Badly decayed teeth requiring extensive restorative dentistry should be extracted, jagged alveolar ridges smoothed and the overlying gingival mucosa gently sutured and allowed to heal before treatment commences. In the past, extraction of all teeth within the beam or even full mouth extractions were considered proper, but are no longer considered necessary. Once the patient has begun treatment, a program of gentle but thorough oral hygiene should be enforced. Fluoride gels have proven to be extremely helpful in preventing subsequent dental caries. Patients apply the gel to flexible holders which keep the gel in contact with the teeth for a few minutes per day. In this manner the M. D. Anderson Hospital Group[7] was able to decrease post-irradiation caries from about 65 to 30%. Keys and McCasland[9] reported a similar program which resulted in fewer extractions, fewer clinic visits and 75% fewer cavities after irradiation.

Recently saliva substitutes have become available. Shannon *et* al.[10,11] have described a new product which not only lubricates the mouth, thereby ameliorating xerostomia, but also helps remineralize enamel of the teeth.

Lung. Although radiation induced pulmonary damage occurs at moderate doses, it usually does not present a substantial risk to the patient, because it is confined to the treated portal. Surrounding normal lung frequently can compensate for the loss of function in the damaged lung. In contrast, chemotherapy induced damage affects the entire pulmonary parenchyma. Fortunately it is quite rare.

Libshitz and Southard[12] provide a review of pulmonary complications secondary to radiotherapy. In most cases, two distinct phases of damage, characterized by pneumonitis and fibrosis, are seen; however, either can, at times, occur by itself. Initially inflammatory type changes arise approximately 2 months after completion of treatment. Patients may complain of cough or dyspnea and a chest x ray may show changes ranging from a slight haze to a dense alveolar infiltrate; however, correlation between the patient's symptoms and x ray changes not infrequently is poor. Patients who are markedly symptomatic may have minimal radiographic findings and vice versa. Within a few months of treatment, the previously described pneumonitis usually transforms into fibrosis. While radiation induced fibrosis is identical in composition and symptomatology to fibrosis of any etiology, diagnosis of radiation-induced fibrosis usually can be made unequivocally on the basis of x-ray findings. The well-defined spatial pattern precisely corresponds to the treatment portal, not to an anatomic boundary, and stabilizes by 9 to 12 months after treatment, whereas recurrent tumor progresses unceasingly.

Pulmonary toxicity secondary to chemotherapy has been reviewed by Schein and Winokur.[13] Such changes are encountered with busulfan and bleomycin although cases secondary to methotrexate treatment have been reported. As with radiation induced damage, dose appears to be a critical factor. Patients who receive busulfan for prolonged periods may develop a subtle, progressive syndrome of cough, dyspnea and low grade fever, years after initiation of therapy. Chest x rays reveal both intra-alveolar and interstitial infiltrates, and pulmonary function studies show restrictive lung disease and poor diffusing capacity. Because these changes are non-specific, neoplastic involvement of lung or an infectious etiology needs to be ruled out and may require a diagnostic biopsy which will reveal only chronic pneumonitis and pulmonary fibrosis. Thus, the histologic picture of "busulfan lung" is similar to that seen after pulmonary irradiation. Unfortunately, once established, busulfan lung is fatal within 6 months of diagnosis in the majority of cases, despite withdrawal of drug and administration of corticosteroids.

Pulmonary changes secondary to bleomycin produce the drug's dose limiting toxicity. Clinically these changes are manifest as a non-productive cough or dyspnea. Radiographs show diffuse interstitial fibrosis and patchy basal infiltrates. Pulmonary function tests reveal restrictive lung disease and decreased diffusing capacity. Biopsy characteristically reveals a pattern of diffuse fibrosis similar to that seen with busulfan. Treatment again consists of withdrawal of drug and administration of steroids.

In contrast, pulmonary changes secondary to methotrexate appear to occur on an allergic basis. Within a few weeks of initiation of therapy (and unrelated to the total dose) the patient experiences the abrupt onset of fever, a non-productive cough, and dyspnea. Chest x-rays reveal patchy intra-alveolar and interstitial infiltrates and a biopsy reveals infiltration of the lung by lymphocytes, giant cells and non-caseating granulomas. Within a few days after withdrawal of the drug, resolution occurs. Steroids may hasten this process.

Heart. Although changes in electrocardiographic patterns have been noted as a result of irradiation of the heart, direct damage to the myocardium is not a clinical concern with doses in common practice. On the other hand, damage to the pericardial covering and perhaps to the coronary arteries may present management problems. Stewart et al.[14] reviewed the records of patients who had received elective irradiation for breast carcinoma or therapeutic irradiation for malignant lymphoma and found an incidence of pericardial damage of approximately 5%. In most cases, complications arose between 6 months and 4 years after therapy and consisted either of acute pericarditis (with or without effusion) or chronic constrictive pericarditis. Even when pericardial effusion occurs, most patients recover. Simple anti-inflammatory medication usually suffices as treatment; however, it is important to rule out effusion secondary to *recurrent* disease which requires more aggressive therapy. Should the effusion prove unresponsive, a pericardial window may have to be considered. Constrictive pericarditis may necessitate pericardiectomy.

Non-specific electrocardiographic changes have been noted coincident with administration of chemotherapeutic drugs. However, like radiotherapy induced changes, they seem to be of no clinical importance. In contrast, progressive cardiac failure secondary to cardiomyopathy also has been associated with administration of these drugs. Lefrak, Pitha and Rosenheim[15] reported data concerning nearly 400 patients who received doxorubicin (adriamycin) and found that, when total doses were *less* than 500 mg per square meter of body surface, congestive failure was extremely rare. In contrast, when the total dose exceeded this figure, 30% of patients went on to manifest cardiac failure. Halazun et al.[16] found similar cardiac toxicity in children treated with daunorubicin for acute lymphocytic leukemia. Because of this type of toxicity, these drugs should not be used at doses above 500 mg per square meter of body surface. However, even then subclinical cardiac damage may predispose the patient to future problems. For example, Friedman et al.[17] found endomyocardial damage by serial biopsy after as little as 180 mg per square meter of adriamycin.

In addition, concern about *the possibility* of treatment induced coronary artery occlusion may be warranted. Fajardo and Stewart[18] reported coronary artery disease in patients who received radiotherapy. Kopelson and Herwig[19] reported myocardial infarction associated with chemotherapy. While such anecdotal reports clearly do not prove the case, they do imply that treatment may have a deleterious effect upon the patency of the coronary arteries. More precise estimation of the risk, however, is precluded by the occurrence of similar findings, secondary to tumor itself.

Liver. In 1965, Ingold et al.[20] carefully described hepatic damage secondary to irradiation. If tolerance is exceeded, approximately 1 month after treatment the liver becomes enlarged, the patient gains weight and may begin to experience abdominal pain or ascites. Chemical abnormalities (most reliably an elevated alkaline phosphatase level) also occur. Liver scans utilizing radiocolloids will fail to demonstrate uptake in the irradiated area and, unlike metastatic disease, the defect conforms to the shape of the irradiated portal. Although rarely necessary, a liver biopsy at this stage would show typical histologic changes, primarily in the centrolobular region, consisting of congestion of sinusoids, hyperemia and hemorrhage with atrophy of hepatic cells. Therapy is basically supportive, consisting of bed rest and a high protein, high calorie diet, but, in essence, the patient must be able to recover on his own, implying that, if at all possible, some portion of the liver from which regeneration can occur should be left unirradiated. Even if the patient does recover, fibrosis, particularly of periportal areas, will occur in time. This has been taken as evidence by some that the mechanism of radiation induced damage is via destruction of fine vasculature rather than direct hepatocellular death.

Hepatic toxicity of chemotherapy is well established for methotrexate and 6-mercaptopurine. The use of methotrexate in non-neoplastic diseases has permitted study of subsequent changes over prolonged periods, without the complicating influence of liver metastases. Toxicity of methotrexate appears to result from repeated hepatic damage by the drug. Interestingly, toxicity is less related to total dose than to persistant hepatic insult; frequent small doses produced significantly more damage than intermittent large doses.[21-23] Histopathologic changes secondary to administration of methotrexate consist primarily of cirrhosis and hepatic fibrosis developing in 20 to 30% of patients treated for prolonged periods. Unfortunately, although one would hope to detect these changes in an early phase, liver function blood chemistry tests appear to be inadequate for this purpose. When prolonged administration of methotrexate is deemed advisable, some authors recommend percutaneous liver biopsies on a regular basis for detection of early toxicity.

Hepatic toxicity secondary to 6-mercaptopurine appears to occur on a different basis. To begin with, damage begins more rapidly after initiation of therapy, frequently within 1 to 2 months and, histopathologically, is characterized by hepatocellular necrosis and biliary stasis. In contrast to methotrexate, changes can be monitored by liver chemistries, manifestations of toxicity frequently producing elevation in serum transaminase levels. Last, these abnormalities spontaneously revert to normal after cessation of therapy. While the incidence of hepatic toxicity is difficult to measure precisely, jaundice developing in association with therapy for acute leukemia has been reported in 10 to 40% of patients.[24,25]

Kidney. Radiation induced renal damage has been reviewed by Aron and Schlesinger.[26] Both acute and chronic radiation induced nephritis occur, the former potentially life threatening, the latter compatible with prolonged life.

Acute radiation nephritis usually develops after a latent period of 6 months to 1 year producing hypertension (of variable degree) and uremia. Patients may complain of edema, dyspnea, headaches, nocturia, vomiting and generalized weakness. Urinalysis reveals albuminuria and inappropriately dilute urine. Hematuria is unusual. Although the level of hypertension does not appear to influence the patient's prognosis, elevation of blood urea nitrogen level above 100 mg per 100 ml is ominous. At this stage, biopsy shows widespread damage to the glomeruli and tubules plus interstitial fibrosis between tubules. Once established, the disease may regress but never completely remits. Eventually chronic radiation nephritis develops.

Chronic radiation induced nephritis is characterized by proteinuria, anemia and azotemia. Hypertension, if present, generally is of a lesser degree than is seen in acute nephritis. In several ways changes resemble chronic glomerulonephritis, biopsy principally revealing glomerular damage, although secondary tubular fibrosis and atrophy can also be found. Serial intravenous urograms will demonstrate progressive shrinkage of the affected kidney as is seen in many types of end stage renal disease.

Renal damage secondary to chemotherapy occurs rarely. The most specific toxin is the drug streptozotocin whose dose limiting toxicity is renal tubular damage. The precise time course and total dose required to produce this change appears to be quite variable, and fortunately, the typical early manifestation of proteinuria appears to be reversible within a month of discontinuance of therapy. Should therapy not be discontinued or high doses of the drug be given, the patient may develop azotemia and death may ensue.[27,28]

DeFronzo et al.[29] have described renal toxicity in association with high dose cyclophosphamide therapy characterized by impaired water excretion. Clinically the patients become hyponatremic, have decreased urinary volume and inappropriately concentrated urine. Apparently, these changes result from the action of metabolites of the drug on the distal renal tubule, and the change is reversible if the drug is withheld.

Bladder. Radiation induced bladder complications basically occur secondary to alterations in the microvasculature. Fibrosis, endarteritis and telangiectasia may all contribute to relative ischemia which, in turn, leads to atrophy or necrosis manifested by ulcers or fistulas. Because of the time required for vascular changes to occur, radiation induced complications typically present a year or more after treatment. Hemorrhagic cystitis without a specific bleeding site may also occur. When conservative therapy is not successful, instillation of dilute formalin solutions may provide relief. In severe cases, cystectomy may be necessary. Ulceration may heal with conservative measures and adequate hygiene to prevent superinfection. Vesicovaginal or vesicorectal fistulas secondary to aggressive therapy of large cervical tumors generally are not repaired. The only possible treatment for such fistulas is surgical.

Chemotherapy induced bladder damage occurs with cyclophosphamide. In many ways, this damage is similar to that produced by irradiation, characterized by telangiectasia, edema and fibrosis. The change appears to be dose related and as many as one-quarter of patients who receive long term treatment with cyclophosphamide can be shown to have bladder fibrosis at autopsy.[30] As also occurs in irradiated bladders, telangiectatic vessels are extremely fragile and hemorrhagic cystitis can occur with little provocation. Treatment includes withdrawal of drug and management as outlined under radiation induced changes.

Gastrointestinal Tract. Radiation induced damage can occur in any part of the alimentary tract, each producing individual symptomatology and requiring specific therapy.[31]

With moderate dose levels, irradiation-induced damage of the stomach is uncommon; however, epigastric pain, bleeding and vomiting may occur approximately 1 to 2 months after treatment. A gastrointestinal x-ray series may then reveal a lesion often appearing identical to a classic peptic ulcer. Affected patients should be placed on a strict medical regimen, as is typically used for peptic ulceration secondary to other etiologies, and, with such treatment, healing frequently occurs within 2 to 3 months. If damage has been so intense that healing does not follow treatment, partial gastrectomy may become necessary; however, such procedures should not be undertaken lightly because of risk of small bowel damage.

The small intestine, in particular the duodenum, is the most radioresponsive gastrointestinal structure. Acute small intestinal complications frequently present as an "acute abdomen," including severe pain, nausea, vomiting, distention and, at times, bloody diarrhea. Sometimes a pseudotumor mass may be palpated. An x ray reveals distended loops of small and large bowel with characteristic air-fluid interfaces. Appropriate management consists of decompression and laparotomy if a perforated ulcer or infarction is suspected. Surgical management must be individualized, but as a general rule, the most limited surgical procedure that produces relief should be used.

Chronic small intestinal damage generally results from vascular changes. The functional integrity of the intestine is markedly diminished and malabsorption of carbohydrates, proteins, fats and fluid becomes a substantial problem. A GI x-ray series reveals stenosed, ulcerated or dilated loops of bowel which can simulate recurrent disease or non-neoplastic etiologies such as Crohn's disease.

The large intestine and rectum are less responsive to irradiation than the small intestine. Consequently, complications in this area usually are seen only when localized high-dose therapy is delivered to the recto-sigmoid region, generally during treatment of cervical carcinoma. Within 6 months to 3 years of treatment, the patient may complain of blood in the stool, diarrhea or tenesmus. An x ray reveals stenosis and/or ulceration. Management should initially be aimed at decreasing irritation in the region by low residue, soft diets. When pain is the prime complaint, topical steroid preparations may be helpful. For severe problems not ameliorated by conservative management, a diverting colostomy may be necessary.

While dose and volume irradiated are prime determinants of risk for the GI tract, the risk is intensified if mobility is impaired. Consequently, patients who have had previous abdominal surgery, and whose risk of adhesions is, therefore, substantial, must be considered at greater risk for the previously described complications.

Gastrointestinal complications secondary to chemotherapy rarely occur. The most common is mediated through the previously described neurotoxicity of vincristine (Chap. 16) wherein patients develop paralytic ileus. In such cases the drug should be withheld and nasogastric tube decompression ordered.

References

1. Kramer, S.: The Hazards of Therapeutic Irradiation of the Central Nervous System. Clin. Neurosurg. *15*:301–318, 1968.
2. Kramer, S. and Lee, K.F.: Complication of Radiation Therapy: the Central Nervous System. Semin. Roentgenol. *9*:75–83, 1974.
3. Merriam, G.R. and Focht, E.F.: A Clinical Study of Radiation Cataracts and the Relationship to Dose. A.J.R. *77*:759–785, 1957.
4. Shukovsky, L.J. and Fletcher, G.H.: Retinal and Optic Nerve Complications in a High Dose Irradiation Technique of Ethmoid Sinus and Nasal Cavity. Radiology *104*:629–634, 1972.
5. Rubin, P. and Casarett, G.W.: *Clinical Radiation Pathology*, Philadelphia, W.B. Saunders Co., 1968, p. 561.
6. MacComb, W.S.: Necrosis in Treatment of Intraoral Cancer by Radiation Therapy. A.J.R. *87*:431–440, 1962.
7. Daly, T.E., Drane, J.B. and MacComb, W.S.: Management of Problems of the Teeth and Jaw in Patients Undergoing Irradiation. Am. J. Surg. *124*:539–542, 1972.
8. Dreizen, S., *et al.*: Oral Complications of Cancer Radiotherapy. Postgrad. Med. *61*:85–92, 1977.
9. Keys, H.M. and McCasland, J.P.: Techniques and Results of a Comprehensive Dental Care Program in Head and Neck Cancer Patients. Int. J. Radiat. Oncol., Biol. Phys. *1*:859–865, 1976.
10. Shannon, I.L., McCrary, B.R., and Starcke, E.N.: A Saliva Substitute for Use by Xerostomic Patients Undergoing Radiotherapy to the Head and Neck. Oral Surg. *44*:656–661, 1977.

11. Shannon, I.L., Trodahl, J.N., and Starcke, E.N.: Remineralization of Enamel by a Saliva Substitute Designed for Use by Irradiated Patients. Cancer 41:1746–1750, 1978.
12. Libshitz, H.I. and Southard, M.E.: Complications of Radiation Therapy: the Thorax. Semin. Roentgenol. 9:41–49, 1974.
13. Schein, P.S. and Winokur, S.H.: Immunosuppressive and Cytoxic Chemotherapy: Long-term Complications. Ann. Intern. Med. 82:84–95, 1975.
14. Stewart, J.R., et al.: Radiation-induced Heart Disease. Radiology 89:302–310, 1967.
15. Lefrak, E.A., Pitha, J. and Rosenheim, S.: A Clinicopathologic Analysis of Adriamycin Cardiotoxicity. Cancer 32:302–314, 1973.
16. Halazun, J.F., et al.: Daunorubicin Cardiac Toxicity in Children with Acute Lymphocytic Leukemia. Cancer 33:545–554, 1974.
17. Friedman, M.A., et al.: Doxorubicin Cardiotoxicity. J.A.M.A. 240:1603–1606, 1978.
18. Fajardo, L.F. and Stewart, J.R.: Coronary Artery Disease after Irradiation. N. Engl. J. Med. 286:1265–1266, 1972.
19. Kopelson, G. and Herwig, K.J.: The Etiologies of Coronary Artery Disease in Cancer Patients. Int. J. Radiat. Oncol., Biol. Phys. 4:895–906, 1978.
20. Ingold, J.A., et al.: Radiation Hepatitis. A.J.R. 93:200–208, 1965.
21. Dahl, M.G.C., Gregory, M.M. and Scheuler, P.J.: Methotrexate Hepatotoxicity in Psoriasis—Comparison of Different Dose Regimens. Br. Med. J. 1:654–656, 1972.
22. Cooperative Study: Psoriasis - Liver - Methotrexate Interactions. Arch. Dermatol. 108:36–42, 1973.
23. Tobias, H. and Auerbach, R.: Hepatotoxicity of Long-term Methotrexate Therapy for Psoriasis. Arch. Intern. Med. 132:391–396, 1973.
24. McIlvanie, S.K. and MacCarthy, J.D.: Hepatitis in Association with Prolonged 6-Mercaptopurine Therapy. Blood 14:80–90, 1959.
25. Einborn, M. and Davidsohn, I.: Hepatotoxicity of Mercaptopurine. J.A.M.A. 188:802–806, 1964.
26. Aron, B.S. and Schlesinger, A.: Complications of Radiation Therapy: the Genitourinary Tract. Semin. Roentgenol. 9:65–74, 1974.
27. Sadoff, L.: Nephrotoxicity of Streptozotocin. Cancer Chemotherapy Rep. 54:457–459, 1970.
28. Schein, P.S., et al.: Clinical Antitumor Activity and Toxicity of Streptozotocin. Cancer 34:993–1000, 1974.
29. DeFronzo, R.A., et al.: Water Intoxication in Man after Cyclophosphamide Therapy. Ann. Intern. Med. 78:861–869, 1973.
30. Johnson, W.W. and Meadows, D.C.: Urinary Bladder Fibrosis and Telangiectasia Associated with Long-term Cyclophosphamide Therapy. N. Engl. J. Med. 284:290–294, 1971.
31. Roswit, B.: Complications of Radiation Therapy: the Alimentary Tract. Semin. Roentgenol. 9:51–63, 1974.

18

EFFECTS ON
REPRODUCTION

To a greater or lesser degree, the gonads are affected by all methods of non-surgical cancer therapy. Even if gonadal tissue is not directly within an irradiated volume, some radiations may be scattered from structures that are within the treatment volume and absorbed in the gonads. The amount of radiation received by the gonads under such circumstances may range from exceedingly small to relatively substantial and vary according to the type of equipment used and the distance between treatment volume and gonads. Radiation intensity always decreases as a function of distance, because many radiations are absorbed in the material between the source and object of interest (in this case the gonads). Certainly, if gonads are directly irradiated during therapy (i.e. they cannot somehow be shielded), large doses may be absorbed in them, sufficient to cause considerable damage.

Systemic administration of chemotherapeutic drugs may result in damaging doses being received by many normal tissues of the body, and gonads are no exception. In fact, gonadal tissue may be among the most vulnerable to damage because of the relatively high rate of proliferative activity of its cells.

Sterility and Impaired Fertility—Radiation. High doses of radiation unquestionably impair fertility and may even cause sterility. Precursor cells to mature sperm and ova are radiosensitive and may be killed by treatment so that no *new* sperm can be produced or ova matured. Mature sperm and ova present at the time of irradiation are not always killed by doses received during radiotherapy, because, compared to their precursors, they are resistant. Any impairment of fertility would not become evident until some time after irradiation, when whatever supply of mature sperm or ova is exhausted.

The difference between impaired fertility and sterility appears to be one of degree. Radiation can be absorbed in gonads without killing *all* precursor cells to mature gametes, but greatly reducing their number. When this happens, the production of new gametes may not fall to zero, but can be greatly reduced. Since the *probability* of fertilization depends on numbers, oligospermia or reduced numbers of ova greatly reduces that probability, but may not reduce it to zero.

In the clinical sense, the production of sterility requires single radiation exposures approximately double the size of a single fraction commonly used in radiation therapy (about 400 rad). If the gonads are within an irradiated volume and cannot be shielded, that dose (and greater) can easily be absorbed, but not ordinarily in a single fraction. However, over a few fractions an *equivalent* dose may be accumulated and sterility may result.

If gonads are not in the treated field but absorb only scattered radiation, substantial doses are unlikely to accumulate and sterility is unlikely to occur, although impaired fertility is not impossible.

Sterility and Impaired Fertility—Chemotherapy. Chemotherapeutic agents also cause impairment of fertility and sterility in both men and women.[1-22] In men, conventional doses of chlorambucil[7,8,18] or cyclophosphamide[13-15,17] and combination chemotherapy using chlorambucil and cyclophosphamide;[19] cyclophosphamide, vincristine and prednisone (CVP, COP); nitrogen mustard, vincristine, procarbazine and prednisone (MOPP); or nitrogen mustard, vincristine, methotrexate and prednisone (MOMP)[21] have all proved to produce aspermia, oligospermia and/or testicular atrophy. Sterility or impaired fertility was not always irreversible[19] and spermatogenesis returned in a few cases.

The effect on the immature testis is less clear. Some authors have found an adverse action of chemotherapy on spermatogenesis, but others[11] showed none. Possibly, the time relative to puberty that treatment is given is important;[20] *early* puberty may be sensitive to the action of chemotherapeutic drugs but *later* puberty, less so.

In women, chemotherapeutic drugs may cause amenorrhea and suppression of ovarian function. Cyclophosphamide[5,6,9,10,16] clearly has been implicated, and the effects usually are irreversible.[14] In women treated with combination drug therapy for Hodgkin's disease, amenorrhea or severe oligomenorrhea has been noted after vinblastine, nitrogen mustard and chlorambucil; nitrogen mustard and chlorambucil; nitrogen mustard, vinblastine, vincristine and procarbazine; or vinblastine and cyclophosphamide combinations.[10] A dose response relationship has been reported[16] with chlorambucil, vinblastine and procarbazine combinations; amenorrhea did not occur in some patients receiving low doses.

Women treated for leukemia with busulfan have experienced amenorrhea and ovarian suppression.[1,2] Thus, it is fair to say that cytotoxic agents, especially the alkylating agents, have deleterious effects on female fertility. There may be some dose dependence to the effect and it may depend to an extent on the length of time of treatment. The antifertility effects sometimes may be reversible, but when so, usually revert only *partly*, many months after treatment is over.

Congenital Defects. The question frequently arises: Does irradiation or exposure of the gonads to chemotherapeutic drugs result in malformations of children conceived *after* cessation of either radiation or chemotherapy? If this were to occur, it would be an important complication of non-surgical treatment of young people. LeFloch et al.[23] found no abnormalities in 8 babies born to 6 women who were treated for Hodgkin's disease by radiotherapy, with or without chemotherapy. Holmes and Holmes[24] reported no impairment of fertility or developmental abnormalities that could be attributed to treatment in 68 pregnancies of 35 patients who received only irradiation for Hodgkin's disease. However, 21 pregnancies in 13 other patients who were treated by both chemotherapy and irradiation produced a significantly higher rate of spontaneous abortions and abnormal offspring. In other studies methotrexate and actinomycin-D therapy had no effect either on morbidity or birth defects among pregnancies conceived after treatment ended,[25] and neither did chemotherapy of young girls for leukemia,[26] but children born to two fathers treated for acute myelogenous leukemia with cytosine arabinoside and daunorubicin were severely deformed.[27] Such a small body of evidence, however, is difficult to interpret and no firm conclusions can be drawn.

Effects on the Gene Pool. Both ionizing radiations and many of the drugs used in chemotherapy of cancer are mutagenic. Since this is so, the therapeutic use of these agents in human beings raises the possibility that they will damage human genetic material in a way that can be transmitted to future generations.

Because non-surgical therapy can increase the frequency with which mutations occur and because detrimental mutations outweigh beneficial mutations in terms of numbers, there is a possibility that treatment could damage the aggregate genetic material of the human race by increasing its burden of detrimental mutations. While this possibility cannot and should not be dismissed lightly, careful evaluation suggests it is not a serious problem, at least not at present. For the most part, persons who get and are treated for cancer are beyond reproductive age. Any mutation produced in their gonads has little chance of entering the gene pool because so few become parents. While young people sometimes do require anticancer therapy, its relative infrequency insures that the number of mutations placed in the gene pool this way is small. The impact of this small number of mutations on the gene pool is probably small.

Effects on Progeny. It is possible that progeny of persons whose gonads have been affected by non-surgical treatment will abort (or die shortly after birth) or exhibit congenital abnormalities. However, the more likely way for such disasters to occur is if a fetus is directly exposed to anticancer therapy.

Intrauterine life is a period of great sensitivity. Agents producing only mild effects in postnatal life may produce profound changes in the developing embryo or fetus. Thus, it should come as no surprise that both ionizing radiations and some of the drugs used as cancer chemotherapies have been shown to be capable of altering fetal development. The question dealt with in the remainder of this chapter is whether radiations or chemotherapeutic drugs *as they are used therapeutically* affect fetal development.

Embryonic and Fetal Sensitivity. Embryonic and fetal sensitivity apparently stems from three characteristics: (1) During intrauterine life many cells are dividing rapidly, (2) differentiation of these cells is occurring and (3) embryos and fetuses are composed of relatively few cells which must give rise to the large number of cells in the adult body. Consider each of these separately. As has already been described (Chaps. 7 and 8), proliferating cells are more sensitive to radiation and to many chemotherapeutic agents than are quiescent ones. Therefore, it follows that embryos and fetuses with their large proportion of proliferating cells would be more radio- and chemosensitive than later stages of life.

Second, although reasons for this are not known, the process of *differentiation* appears to confer radiosensitivity upon cells.

However, the principal reason for the extraordinarily sensitivity of the unborn, is probably the third, the fact that early life forms are composed of few cells. Since each embryonic or fetal cell gives rise to many adult ones, the loss of a few can result in failure of genesis of large segments of the adult body. Exactly when irradiation or drug damage occurs, determines the type and extent of damage.

Preimplantation. After fertilization, but prior to implantation in the uterus approximately 10 days later, the fertilized egg undergoes repeated cell division but does not enlarge, going from a single large cell (the fertilized ovum) to a structure of the same size consisting of several hundred cells. However, each of these small cells is more-or-less alike. That is, each appears to have about the same *potential* as the fertilized ovum, the potential to produce an entire organism.

Damage at the preimplantation stage, resulting in cell loss, usually produces one of two results. If enough cells are killed, the embryo dies, and there is an early abortion. On the other hand, even if some cells are killed, the embryo may survive. Should that occur, there is a good chance a child will be born that is normal—at least with respect to structure, size and weight—because the remaining cells have the potential to produce an entire new organism.

Organogenesis. Shortly after implantation, the process of organogenesis begins. The undifferentiated embryo differentiates into primitive germ layers (entoderm, ectoderm and mesoderm), and from these, organs differentiate. Damage resulting in cell loss during this period is less likely to produce abortion than during the previous period, because the embryo now is composed of many cells, and loss of some of them no longer is critical. On the other hand, damage resulting in the loss of cells, is likely to result in abnormalities of development. Organs may not be properly or fully formed, but unless the structural deficit is in a vital organ and very great, embryonic or fetal death is not likely.

Organogenesis takes place over several weeks, but the early part of it between 20 and 40 days after conception seems most critical. Damage resulting in cell loss during this period, if it causes any effects at all, is most likely to produce congenital deformities or death at or shortly after birth. (While individuals can survive severe abnormalities in the protected environment of the uterus, often they cannot do so as an independent entity.)

Growth. After organogenesis, the developing embryo grows rapidly for the remainder of intrauterine life. Insults resulting in cell loss during this period have a relatively small chance of causing fetal death; the fetus is composed of many cells and the loss of some, usually is not vital. Also, such insults have a small chance of producing developmental abnormalities, because the new organs also consist of many cells and the loss of a few of them does not result in *detectable* abnormalities in the structure or size of organs.

If any effect is to be observed from insults resulting in cell loss, what is likely to occur is the birth of small but well-formed babies. Growth retardation, if not too severe, can be made up during childhood and adolescence, but if very severe, may result in a small adult.

Intrauterine Death. Both irradiation[28] and chemotherapeutic drugs[29-32] produce intrauterine death. The most probable time in gestation for this to occur is in the preimplantation period; the smallest doses may cause it then. Naturally, by using a high enough dose, embryos or fetuses can be killed at any time in development.

Congenital Malformation from Radiation Therapy. Clear evidence of increased incidence of congenital malformations from radiation therapy for malignant disease is difficult to find, because the number of instances in which pregnant women have received radiation therapy are few. It is known that following exposure of the fetus to *high* doses of radiation, the probability of a severely malformed child is quite high;[33] however, save for circumstances in which the fetus unknowingly is included in the irradiated volume, such doses are unlikely to occur. It is difficult to predict with any degree of certainty the probability of occurrence of malformation after lower doses. In part, this difficulty stems from the belief that a malformation will occur only if several cells, at least, are killed or made non-proliferative during organogenesis. The loss of a single cell at this stage is considered unlikely to result in a *grossly* malformed organ. Because several cells must be killed or sterilized to result in gross malformation, the possibility exists that small doses of radiation do not produce malformations. A threshold dose of radiation *conceivably* could exist below which malformations do not occur although, if any in fact exists, it probably would vary among various individuals and most likely would change as embryonic development progressed. Early in organogenesis, the loss of a few cells might well result in a deformity; the loss of the cells' descendants leaving a major deficit in the mature organ. Later in organogenesis, once the organ consists of many cells, the loss of a few might leave no detectable deficit. To produce substantial deficit might then require the death of many cells and a correspondingly higher radiation dose would be required.

Because high doses to the embryo or fetus produce high probabilities of fetal death or severe abnormalities, direct irradiation of the fetus is unacceptable. Doses of radiation absorbed by the fetus during therapy, therefore, are usually the result of scatter and are small. Consequently, it is not possible to predict accurately the probability of fetal malformations resulting from them. Insufficient human data exist in these dose ranges to draw any conclusions, and it is hard to be sure if animal data can be extrapolated. Many authorities agree, however, that small doses on the order of 10 rad or less have no *practical* expectation of producing gross malformations.[34-36] Even doses two and one-half times as high, may be relatively "safe" from the point of view of abnormality production, at least in the view of some experts.[34] Nevertheless, irradiation of pregnant women requires evaluation of the benefits and risks of treatment, the benefits accruing principally to the mother, but the risks being principally of the unborn.

Congenital Malformation from Chemotherapy. Many antineoplastic drugs exert embryotoxic and/or teratogenic effects in animals. In humans, there is little data, but at least some children born to mothers receiving chemotherapy for cancer have been severely malformed.[29-32,37-39] These effects, in humans, have been noted when the drugs were given during the first trimester; few have been reported in the second and third trimesters. However, human data *are* scanty. Chlorambucil,[37] cyclophosphamide[38] and aminopterin[39] have already been implicated but other drugs may well produce similar changes. Thus, in light of the multiple and severe congenital abnormalities that have been produced by chemotherapy, we believe that the presence of a fetus, at least in its first trimester, should be considered a strong contraindication to the use of chemotherapy. Conversely, if chemotherapy is deemed essential in a pregnant woman, in particular in the first trimester, therapeutic abortion must be considered as an alternative to the substantial probability of producing a deformed child.

Fetal Growth. Once organogenesis is complete, the most probable effect of radiotherapy or chemotherapy is retarded growth of the developing fetus and small babies have been observed among the survivors of the atomic explosions at Hiroshima and Nagasaki. Approximately 40 rad or more appears to be necessary to increase the incidence of small babies;[34] insufficient human data concerning chemotherapy exist to make any dose related predictions.

Treatment Resulting in Cell Injury. Thus far, only *lethal* cellular injury has been discussed, however, depending on various factors, chief among them dose, embryonic or fetal cells may not be killed by an insult. Instead they may be sub-lethally but irreversibly damaged. If this occurs—and these damaged cells retain their ability to proliferate—a subpopulation of cells could be produced within affected organisms, carrying the unrepaired defect. One possible expression of such a defect is cancer. Irradiation or treatment with carcinogenic chemotherapeutic agents *in utero* has some probability of causing a tumor to arise subsequently. Two aspects should be noted: (1) the particular type of cancer induced will depend on the embryonic or fetal tissue exposed, and (2) the dose of either drug or radiation must be sufficiently *low* to produce this *sublethal* effect. Concerning the former: Irradiation early in pregnancy almost inevitably exposes the total embryo or fetus. During the first trimester the baby is small and if the pelvis is irradiated, the probability is that all, or nearly all, of the fetus will be included. Even if the pelvis is not directly irradiated, the fetus nevertheless may be exposed to radiations scattered from structures (particularly bone) in the irradiated field. Under these conditions, too, early fetuses are likely to be irradiated totally, although the exposure may not be uniform over all parts of the fetal body.

When the entire body is irradiated, one may expect the most sensitive part to respond first. In theory, at least, this would be primitive bone marrow so the kind of malignancy *expected* to appear first and most commonly would be leukemia. Irradiation during the first trimester, then, should increase the incidence of leukemia. Although malignant transformations may be produced in a variety of tissues, affected individuals run a risk of succumbing to the cancer appearing first, with survivors later falling victim to another induced neoplasm. However, since (1) the surviving group would in all probability be small, significant increases in second cancers would be hard to demonstrate and (2) the means of "curing" leukemics (chemotherapy and radiation) are carcinogenic, the task of assigning responsibility for the second neoplasm is formidable.

Chemotherapeutic drugs cross placenta and circulate freely among fetal cells. Because exposure is total body in most cases, they, too, would be expected to induce leukemia primarily. Certain drugs could conceivably accumulate in a given tissue or tissues. If that were to happen, cancers of that tissue might well result. Examples include radioactive sodium-iodide (Iodine-131) which crosses the placenta and, if fetal thyroid is functioning, accumulates in thyroid. The damage caused could result in carcinoma of thyroid later in life. Similarly, diethylstilbestrol (DES) causes gynecologic tract cancers later in the life of girls exposed as fetuses.

The second consideration regarding the probability of induction of cancer in exposed fetuses was dose. Since induction of malignancy is a sublethal cellular effect, cytocidal doses of either radiation or chemotherapeutic agents are not expected to be efficient at increasing cancer incidence. Only low doses are expected to have a reasonable expectation of accomplishing this.

While several studies suggest that embryonic or fetal exposure to diagnostic levels of radiation causes leukemia[10-13] and possibly some non-leukemic cancers, few, if any, report leukemogenesis or carcinogenesis after fetal exposure during radiation therapy. This must be due partly, if not entirely, to what is an extremely small body of experience. Few *pregnant* women receive radiotherapy.

It is also unlikely for the fetus to receive small, potentially leukemogenic or carcinogenic doses of chemotherapeutic agents. The systemic nature of the distribution of these drugs means that they expose the fetus to a dose approximately that received by the mother. Carcinogenesis and/or leukemogenesis is not impossible, but because dose is expected to be high, effects of a different type (abortion, abnormalities of development) are much more likely.

References

1. Louis, J., Limarzi, L.R. and Best, W.R.: Effect of Chlorambucil on Spermatogenesis in the Human with Malignant Lymphoma. Arch. Intern. Med. 97:299–308, 1956.
2. Galton, D.A.G., Till, M. and Wiltshaw, E.: Busulphan (1,4-dimethanesulfonyloxybutane, myleran): Summary of Clinical Results. Ann. N.Y. Acad. Sci. 68:967–973, 1958.
3. Freckman, H.A., et al.: Chlorambucil - Prednisolone Therapy for Disseminated Breast Carcinoma. J.A.M.A. 189:23–26, 1964.
4. Ezdinli, E.E. and Stutzman, L.: Chlorambucil Therapy for Lymphomas and Chronic Lymphocytic Leukemia. J.A.M.A. 190:444–450, 1965.
5. Fosdick, W.M., Parson, J.L. and Hill, D.: Long-term Cyclophosphamide Therapy in Rheumatoid Arthritis. Arthritis Rheum. 11:151–160, 1968.
6. Fries, J.F., et al.: Cyclophosphamide Therapy in Connective Tissue. Clin. Res. 18:134, 1970.
7. Richter, P., et al.: Effect of Chlorambucil on Spermatogenesis in the Human with Malignant Lymphoma. Cancer 25:1026–1030, 1970.

8. Miller, D.G.: Alkylating Agents and Human Spermatogenesis. J.A.M.A. *217*:1662–1665, 1971.
9. Miller, J.J., Williams, G.R. and Leissing, J.C.: Multiple Late Complications of Therapy with Cyclophosphamide, Including Ovarian Destruction. Am. J. Med. *50*:530–535, 1971.
10. Sobrinho, L., Levine, R.A. and DeConti, R.C.: Amenorrhea in Patients with Hodgkin's Disease Treated with Antineoplastic Agents. Am. J. Obstet. Gynecol. *109*:135–139, 1971.
11. Arneil, G.C.: Cyclophosphamide and the Prepubertal Testis. Lancet *2*:1259–1260, 1972.
12. Cameron, J.S. and Ogg, C.S.: Sterility and Cyclophosphamide. Lancet *1*:1174–1175, 1972.
13. Fairley, K.F., Barrie, J.U. and Johnson, W.: Sterility and Testicular Atrophy Related To Cyclophosphamide Therapy. Lancet *1*:568–569, 1972.
14. George, C.R.P. and Evans, R.A.: Infertility after Treatment with Cyclophosphamide. Lancet *1*:840–841, 1972.
15. Kumar, R., *et al.*: Cyclophosphamide and Reproductive Function. Lancet *1*:1212–1214, 1972.
16. Morgenfeld, M.C., *et al.*: Ovarian Lesions due to Cytostatic Agents During the Treatment of Hodgkin's Disease. Surg. Gynecol. Obstet. *134*:826–828, 1972.
17. Qureshi, M.S.A., *et al.*: Cyclophosphamide Therapy and Sterility. Lancet *2*:1290–1291, 1972.
18. Cheviakoff, S., *et al.*: Recovery of Spermatogenesis in Patients with Lymphoma After Treatment with Chlorambucil. J. Reprod. Fertil. *33*:155–157, 1973.
19. Hinkes, E. and Plotkin, D.: Reversible Drug-induced Sterility in a Patient with Acute Leukemia. J.A.M.A. *223*:1490–1491, 1973.
20. Rapola, J., *et al.*: Cyclophosphamide and the Pubertal Testis. Lancet *1*:98–99, 1973.
21. Sherins, R.J. and DeVita, V.T.: Effect of Drug Treatment for Lymphoma on Male Reproductive Capacity: Studies of Men in Remission after Therapy. Ann. Intern. Med. 79:216–220, 1973.
22. Sieber, S.M. and Adamson, R.H.: Toxicity of Antineoplastic Agents in Man: Chromosomal Aberrations, Antifertility Effects, Congenital Malformations and Carcinogenic Potential. Adv. Cancer Res. *22*:57–155, 1975.
23. LeFloch, O., Donaldson, S.S. and Kaplan, J.S.: Pregnancy Following Oophorectomy and Total Nodal Irradiation in Women with Hodgkin's Disease. Cancer *38*:2263–2268, 1976.
24. Holmes, G.E. and Holmes, F.F.: Pregnancy Outcome of Patients Treated for Hodgkin's Disease. Cancer *41*:1317–1322, 1978.
25. Li, F.P. and Jaffe, N.: Progeny of Childhood Cancer Survivors. Lancet *2*:707, 1974.
26. Siris, E.S., Leventhal, B.G. and Vaitukaitis, J.L.: Effects of Childhood Leukemia and Chemotherapy on Puberty and Reproductive Function in Girls. N. Engl. J. Med. *294*:1143–1146, 1976.
27. Russell, J.A. and Powles, R.L.: Conception and Congenital Abnormalities after Chemotherapy of Acute Myelogenous Leukemia in Two Men. Br. Med. J. *1*(6024):1508, 1976.
28. Rugh, R., Wohlfromm, M. and Varma, A.: Low Dose X-ray Effects in the Precleavage Mammalian Zygote. Radiat. Res. *37*:401–412, 1969.
29. Melzer, H.J.: Congenital Anomalies Due to Attempted Abortion with 4-Aminopteroglutamic Acid. J.A.M.A. *161*:1253, 1956.
30. Warkany, J., Beaudry, D.G. and Homstein, S.: Attempted Abortion with Aminopterin (4 Amino-pteroylglutamic acid). Am. J. Disab. Child. *97*:274–281, 1959.

31. Emerson, D.J.: Congenital Malformation Due to Attempted Abortion with Aminopterin. Am. J. Obstet. Gynecol. *84*:356–357, 1962.

32. Shaw, E.B. and Steinbach, H.L.: Aminopterin-induced Fetal Malformation. Am. J. Dis. Child. *115*:477–482, 1962.

33. Dekaban, A.S.: Abnormalities in Children Exposed to X-radiation During Various Stages of Gestation: Tentative Timetable of Radiation Injury to the Human Fetus. Part I. J. Nuclear Med. 9:471, 1968.

34. Brent, R.L. and Gorson, R.O.: Radiation Exposure in Pregnancy. Curr. Probl. Diagn. Radiol. *11*:1, 1972.

35. Rugh, R.: Radiology and the Human Embryo and Fetus. In *Medical Radiation Biology*, G.V. Dalrymple *et al.* (eds), Philadelphia, W.B. Saunders Co., 1973, p. 92.

36. Hammer-Jacobson, E.: Therapeutic Abortion on Account of X-ray Examination During Pregnancy. Danish Med. Bull. 6:113, 1959.

37. Shotton, D. and Monie, I.W.: Possible Teratogenic Effect of Chlorambucil on a Human Fetus. J.A.M.A. *186*:74–75, 1963.

38. Greenberg, L.H. and Tanaka, K.R.: Congenital Anomalies Probably Induced by Cyclophosphamide. J.A.M.A. *188*:423–426, 1964.

39. Thiersch, J.B.: Therapeutic Abortions with a Folic Acid Antagonist, 4 Aminopteroyl-Glutamic Acid (4-Amino p.g.a.) Administered by the Oral Route. Am. J. Obstet. Gynecol. *63*:1298–1304, 1952.

40. Stewart, A., Webb, J. and Hewitt, D.: A Survey of Childhood Malignancies. Br. Med. J. *1*:1495, 1958.

41. Stewart, A. and Kneale, G.W.: Radiation Dose Effects in Relation to Obstetric X-rays and Childhood Cancer. Lancet *1*:1185, 1970.

42. Holford, R.M.: The Relation Between Juvenile Cancer and Obstetric Radiography. Health Physics *28*:153–161, 1975.

43. Mole, R.M.: Internatal Irradiation and Childhood Cancer: Causation or Coincidence. Br. J. Cancer *30*:199, 1974.

Carcinogenesis, by definition, results from *sublethal* cellular changes; but carcinogenic agents therapeutically are used in doses so large that they become lethal. It may well be that the relative risk of cell killing and potential of cancer induction is a function of dose. At low doses, cellular changes primarily are sublethal and the risk of cancer induction presumably substantial. In contrast, at high doses, damage may be lethal to so many cells that the risk of cells surviving to produce new cancers is small.

Dose, however, is only one factor determining whether an agent will produce lethal or sublethal (including carcinogenic) damage. With respect to ionizing radiation, for example, cellular oxygen tension, the phase in the life cycle and the degree of cellular differentiation, to recall just some of the factors already discussed in this book, all influence the cellular response to any given dose and often can determine whether or not that dose will be lethal.

Influence of Volume. The number of normal tissue cells affected by non-surgical oncologic methods also should influence the relative risk of subsequent cancer induction. In this respect radiation therapy and chemotherapy differ markedly.

With modern teletherapy equipment and well-devised treatment plans, radiation oncologists can deliver relatively high doses, cytocidal to the vast majority of cells within the sharply delimited volume treated. Consequently, the number of cells in which malignant transformation can occur, must be relatively small, because the total number of cells irradiated is limited and a great many of them are killed.

When chemotherapeutic agents are used, the situation differs. Most drugs are distributed throughout the circulation and come into contact with many cells of the body. In addition, the activity of these agents in a given cell often depends upon whether affected cells are in reproductive cycle or not. Antineoplastic agents are effective as cancer therapy when they kill more tumor cells than normal cells. While exploitation of this difference in lethality accounts for the primary success of chemotherapy, it may, in a sense, also account for the possibility of carcinogenesis in normal tissues. The fact that normal tissues are not killed does not mean they have not been injured, and one of the injuries may well be a malignant transformation. Because of the large number of cells in various tissues contacted by chemotherapeutic agents, theoretically at least, a variety of second cancers may result from their use.

Influence of Target Tissue. For any dose delivered or volume exposed, the incidence of induced tumors seems to depend upon the type of tissues exposed. All other factors being equal, second cancers should occur most often in tissues which are vulnerable to sublethal damage and occur first in tissues which have rapid cellular turnover (Chap. 1). By these criteria, bone marrow should be a likely site for induced malignancies to occur. Because the *time* required for cancers to appear after a carcinogen is applied (the length of the latent period for tumor induction) seems to be a function of the degree to which transformed cells are under a stimulus to grow, malignancies may appear more quickly in hemopoietic than in more static, less stimulated tissue.

Of course, for bone marrow to be affected, in such a way as to yield leukemia, a substantial amount must be exposed to the carcinogen. In contrast to chemotherapy, cancer therapy using ionizing radiations rarely exposes much of the body. In general, the field of irradiation can relatively easily be confined to the region of the cancer and little hemopoietic tissue is exposed. There are exceptions, of course; in treating Hodgkin's disease, substantial amounts of the marrow can be irradiated and that sometimes also happens when treating carcinoma of the ovary. But generally, little marrow is exposed so that leukemia would not be expected to be a frequent complication of radiotherapy.

Because of the quantity of marrow exposed and the strong growth stimulus applied to induced cancers of the marrow, one might expect leukemia to be both common and one of the malignancies to occur early following systemic chemotherapy. If leukemias induced by chemotherapy are aggressive and fatal, the carcinogenic action of chemotherapeutic drugs may be limited—as a practical matter—to this malignancy. No other cancers which also may have been induced, will have time to show up. On the other hand, a variety of cancers derived from whatever tissues are in the irradiated field, might result from radiation therapy. These would, in all probability, occur late after therapy, because few adult tissues are active mitotically, resulting in a relatively long latent period for tumor induction.

It remains to be seen how well these theoretical considerations have been borne out by actual observation and to attempt to provide some perspective in evaluating the degree to which carcinogenesis is a hazard of non-surgical oncology.

Radiation Therapy. No reasonable person questions whether exposure to ionizing radiations causes cancer. Ample evidence exists for radiation induction of cancer in a great variety of animals including human beings. A number of general examples suffice to document the point: The survivors of the atomic bomb explosions at Hiroshima and Nagasaki had an elevated incidence of nearly all kinds of cancer compared to the rest of the Japanese population;[1] women who ingested radium in luminous paint applied to the faces of watches later had a variety of cancers, principally those involving bone;[2] physicians using x rays either for diagnosis or therapy contracted skin and hematogenous cancer;[3,4] persons exposed to x rays for radiation therapy of *benign diseases* (examples include treatment of enlarged tonsils, adenoids or thymus, acne, postpartum mastitis and tinea capitis) later demonstrated cancers, evidently induced by the x rays.[5-9]

The question being dealt with here, however, is not whether radiations can induce cancer, but whether radiations *as used for therapy of malignant disease* induces cancer. As yet, no overall, definitive answer is available.

Leukemia. Several recent studies have searched for a relationship between hematologic neoplasia and radiation therapy for Hodgkin's disease or multiple myeloma.[10-12] Such studies were prompted, at least in part, by a number of reports of leukemia in long term survivors of Hodgkin's disease or multiple myeloma who were at the time of diagnosis of leukemia, without evidence of their original disease. No *clear cut* evidence of a significant association was discovered, although some investigators felt radiation therapy could be *implicated* in the appearance of the leukemia. Analysis is complicated by the fact that (1) generally speaking, persons who have one cancer have a relatively high risk of contracting a second,[13] and further, that in particular, Hodgkin's disease and leukemia may naturally be associated,[11] and (2) the number of cases of leukemia arising in Hodgkin's disease and multiple myeloma victims were few, and since there is a possibility of natural association between those diseases and leukemia, no causal relationship could be established between irradiation and the leukemia.

A study seeking a relationship between radiation therapy for ovarian carcinoma and leukemia[14] could find none. Earlier studies of patients who received radiation therapy for a *benign* ovarian disease, metropathia hemorrhagica, did show an increased incidence of leukemia; however, leukemia has not seemed to result from treatment of carcinoma of the ovary. The difference may be that doses used in treating the benign disease were relatively low and carcinogenic, while those used in treatment of carcinoma of the ovary are much higher and largely cytocidal.

Since *statistical* correlations between radiation therapy and leukemia induction, even when therapy has involved considerable amounts of bone marrow, have not been established, leukemia cannot be proved to be a complication of radiation therapy alone. Nevertheless, there are considerable technical difficulties confronting those attempting to study this question, and it may be that, in the future, causal relationships may yet be demonstrated. Still, it seems reasonable to say that, even *if* causal relationships will be shown eventually, the probability of any *given* person contracting a radiation-caused leukemia will be small—although greater than that of an unirradiated person. It does not seem reasonable to suppose that leukemia will be a frequent complication of radiotherapy, at least as it is practiced today. The reason for this conclusion is that, if leukemia were occurring *often* as a result of radiotherapy, studies done so far would have demonstrated it. The difficulties encountered in establishing or rejecting statistical correlations buttress this point. These difficulties stem from the problem of detecting *small* increases against the background of naturally or spontaneously occurring leukemia. Small increases are quite hard to detect. Purely hypothetically, if *all* leukemias reported in current studies to have developed following radiation therapy for another malignancy are accepted as *certainly* having been produced by radiation therapy, the percentage of those treated in whom therapy *induced* leukemia would be less than one half of one percent.

Non-Hematogenous Cancers. There have been occasional reports of non-hematogenous cancers occurring in survivors of other cancers treated by irradiation. Such studies typically involve persons treated 20 or more years ago, who usually were children when treated. D'Angio et al.[15] stated that radiation therapy, as it was practiced 20 to 25 years ago, seems to have caused second malignancies of tissues in the irradiated field. These second, presumably radiation-caused malignancies were not of the mild, easily treated type, but rather were aggressive and frequently fatal. In another study,[16] 414 children treated for cancer were surveyed. Of these a second malignancy occurred in 19, but of these, only 15 could be attributed to prior radiotherapy. Again these were children treated in the mid-1950s so that the cancers induced had a latent period of more than 20 years. The incidence of cancer was much greater than *expected* in the group of 414 children (15 observed/0.7 expected), but the percentage of the group of 414 who got cancer was only 0.036. While there was a great increase over the expected cancer incidence, it must also be clear that the risk incurred by any particular child of contracting a radiation-induced malignancy, within 20 to 25 years was small.

The breakdown of types of cancers which resulted, included the following categories: cancers of bone, thyroid, soft tissue, breast, skin, and acute leukemia. The induced cancers evidently come from any type of tissue in the irradiated field.

There are few reports of radiation therapy induced malignancies in adults. Bone sarcoma induction has been reported[17] after radiation therapy using kilovoltage equipment as the source of therapeutic radiations. While these lesions may represent a *bona fide* complication of young children treated for retinoblastoma, they are a most uncommon post-irradiation neoplasm.

Another group of investigators has reported non-lymphomatous malignant tumors occurring following radiation therapy for Hodgkin's disease and suggests these may be related to the intensity of treatment.[18] A somewhat greater risk of development of second malignancies was seen when radiotherapy was intensive. But the number developing second malignancies following irradiation, even at high intensity, was less than one half of one percent.

Interpretation. Several facts should be stressed bearing on the interpretation of the foregoing information. First, it already has been noted that second, apparently radiation-induced malignancies seem chiefly to have occurred in persons treated as children. This may well relate to the latent period for tumor induction. With radiation carcinogenesis, the latent period typically is long, especially for solid tumors, often in the range of 10 to 40 years. Ten years is the time associated with carcinogenesis in those exposed as children and longer periods are associated with adults. Consequently, a survey going back about 20 years may reveal only those cancers induced in children. Much longer times may well be required before significant increases in cancer incidence in persons treated as adults (if, indeed any will occur) will be manifest. The fact that few or none have been reported to date in adults does not necessarily mean none ever will.

Second, the apparently radiation-induced cancers are the presumed result of radiation therapy given 20 or more years ago. In those days, radiations used were of a type called "kilovoltage," and are not commonly used today. Kilovoltage x rays generally gave higher bone and skin doses, and distribution and localization of dose within the treatment volume was less controlled than currently used ''megavolt-age'' therapy units permit. In addition, because of less precise diagnostic and localizing equipment, treatment volumes themselves may have been somewhat larger than those currently used to treat the same cancers would be. These differences may be quite significant in terms of expected carcinogenesis. Although no one can be sure, one would be reasonable in speculating that current modalities would induce *fewer* cancers than older methods, per treatment.

On the other hand, improved survival may permit the appearance of more cancers than was the case following treatment 20 or 30 years ago. With *more* survivors and longer *survival*, greater numbers of induced cancers could make their appearance. However, considering the overall picture, based on what is known, second malignancies seem to be a rare result of radiation therapy alone, and probably will not be an important or frequent complication in the future.

Chemotherapy. Chemotherapy of cancer has been practiced for a much shorter time than radiation therapy and in consequence there is much less experience on which to draw. Nevertheless, second malignancies following chemotherapy have been reported, but nearly all seem to have been leukemias or multiple myelomas.

Leukemia. There are numerous reports of leukemia, principally though not exclusively acute myelogenous leukemia, following chemotherapy for Hodgkin's disease. We have already called attention to the fact that an association may exist between Hodgkin's lymphoma and leukemia, and this problem complicates analysis of data seeking to establish or reject a link between chemotherapy for Hodgkin's disease and later leukemia. Experience seems to vary. Rosner et al.[10] accumulated from the literature a number of cases of leukemia occurring with or following treatment for Hodgkin's disease. They were not, however, able to establish a *statistically significant* association. In Rosner's survey the majority of patients were not treated by a particular technique or by current standards. A study by Coleman et al.[19] designed to overcome the obstacles presented by lack of systematic and/or outmoded treatment, showed no increase in leukemia in patients treated for Hodgkin's disease with chemotherapeutic agents alone. On the other hand, Toland et al.[20] claim a statistically significant increased risk of leukemia, primarily acute myelogenous, following treatment with drugs.

As time passes and more experience with cancer chemotherapy is accumulated, the risks of chemotherapy for Hodgkin's disease should be known more precisely. However, leukemia should not be considered an *unexpected* event following treatment for Hodgkin's disease (whether this is related to carcinogenicity of treatment, immunosuppressivity of treatment or natural association between the diseases). And, it is likely that the risk of leukemia is related to *intensity* of treatment,[18,20] the more intense the treatment the greater the probability of leukemia.

Leukemia also may result after chemotherapy for cancers other than Hodgkin's disease. There are numerous reports of leukemia following chemotherapy, principally with alkylating agents, for ovarian carcinoma.[21-24] Reimer et al.[25] using historical controls of the National Cancer Institute found 13 cases of non-lymphocytic leukemia among 5455 patients treated with alkylating agents, where 0.62 cases were to be expected. The data showed that the risk of leukemia occurring in patients having ovarian cancer treated by alkylating agents is about 35 times greater in 1-year survivors and about 170 times greater in 2-year survivors, than in victims of ovarian cancer treated in other ways. Again, while a greatly increased, relative risk of leukemia developing in patients treated by alkylating agents exists, the hazard for any given individual, among those treated, is not especially large (consider; 13 out of 5455).

Non-Hematogenous Cancers. Non-hematogenous cancers have been reported following chemotherapy, but the incidence is, at least so far, quite low. Lung, vaginal, breast, urinary bladder, and colon malignancies have been associated with chemotherapy.[20,26] In particular, the drug cyclophosphamide, which has been used to treat a number of different types of primary malignancies including Hodgkin's disease and myeloma, has been noted to lead to secondary tumors of the urinary bladder. The drug tends to be stored in the bladder during excretion and this probably underlies its carcinogenic action in this organ.

In sum, overall, at the present state of knowledge, one can say that second malignancies, principally hematogenous malignancies may occur in low incidence following chemotherapy with alkylating agents. With more time and experience with these and other drugs, a clearer picture may emerge, but for the present it seems that second malignancies are an uncommon complication of chemotherapy, but that the complication rate is related to the intensity of treatment; the more intense, the greater the hazard.

Combined Radiation and Chemotherapy. While the carcinogenic action of radiation and chemotherapy of cancers may be difficult to assess and the rate evidently low, combined radiation and chemotherapy seems clearly to be more carcinogenic. The precise degree of risk reported is not always the same, but varies according to differences in methods used by different institutions and individuals. The careful study by Coleman et al.[19] demonstrated a 2.9 and 3.9% risk of development of leukemia at 5 and 7 years after combined therapy of Hodgkin's disease, compared to a 1.5 and 2.0% risk respectively in victims who did not receive combined therapy. The second neoplasms occurred in patients in clinical remission and the authors see this as a serious complication of the treatment of Hodgkin's disease. There is a growing trend toward combined therapy in many stages of Hodgkin's disease and it is important to be aware of the increased risk of leukemia. Toland et al.[20] also reported considerably higher risks of leukemia in persons treated for Hodgkin's disease with combined modalities, which also was related to the intensity of treatment. The relationship to intensity is confirmed by Coleman et al.[19] Increased risk of non-hematogenous malignant tumors following treatment with combined modalities is also established[18] but there is a lesser risk than of the development of leukemia.

Finally, not all combined chemotherapy and radiation therapy results in greater carcinogenic potential than either alone. D'Angio et al.[15] have shown that actinomycin-D combined with radiation therapy seems to have resulted in decreased carcinogenic risk. They are uncertain of the mechanism but suggest that the combined modalities are quite cytocidal, decreasing the cell population in which malignant transformation is possible.

References

1. Beebe, G.W., Katz, M. and Land, C.E.: Studies on the Mortality of A-bomb Survivors. Mortality and Radiation Dose, 1950–1974. Radiat. Res. 75:138–201, 1978.
2. Rowland, R.E.: Dose and Damage in Long-term Radium Cases. In *Medical Radionuclides: Radiation Dose and Effects*. R.J. Cloutier, C.L. Edwards and W.S. Snyder (eds). AEC conference - 691212, 1970, pp. 369–386.
3. Seltser, R. and Sartwell, P.E.: The Influence of Occupational Exposure to Radiation on the Mortality of American Radiologists and Other Medical Specialties. Am. J. Epidemiol. 81:2–22, 1965.
4. Lewis, E.B.: Leukemia, Multiple Myeloma and Aplastic Anemia in American Radiologists. Science 142:1492, 1963.
5. Hutchinson, G.G.: Late Neoplastic Changes Following Medical Irradiation. Cancer 37:1102–1107, 1976.
6. Hempleman, L.H.: Neoplasms in Persons Treated with X-rays in Infancy: Fourth Survey in 20 Years. J. Nat. Cancer Inst. 55:519–530, 1975.

7. Modan, B., Elaine, R. and Werner, A.: Thyroid Cancer Following Scalp Irradiation. Radiology 123:741–744, 1977.
8. Smith, P.G. and Doll, R.: Late Effects of X Irradiation in Patients Treated for Metropathia Hemorrhagica. Br. J. Radiol. 49:224–232, 1976.
9. Mole, R.H.: The Sensitivity of the Human Breast to Cancer Induction by Ionizing Radiation. Br. J. Radiol. 51:401–405, 1978.
10. Rosner, F. and Grunwald, M.W.: Hodgkin's Disease and Acute Leukemia—Report of Eight Cases and Review of the Literature. Am. J. Med. 57:927–939, 1974.
11. Rosner, F. and Grunwald, H.W.: Multiple Myeloma Terminating in Acute Leukemia—Report of Twelve Cases and Review of the Literature. Am. J. Med. 57:927–939, 1974.
12. Coleman, C.N., et al.: Hematologic Neoplasia in Patients Treated for Hodgkin's Disease. N. Engl. J. Med. 297:1249–1252, 1977.
13. Moertel, C.G.: Incidence and Significance of Multiple Primary Neoplasms. Ann. N.Y. Acad. Sci. 114:886–895, 1964.
14. Reimer, R.R., et al.: Acute Leukemia after Alkylating-Agent Therapy of Ovarian Cancer. N. Engl. J. Med. 297:177–181, 1977.
15. D'Angio, G.J., et al.: Decreased Risk of Radiation-Associated Second Malignant Neoplasms in Actinomycin-D Treated Patients. Cancer 37:1117–1185, 1976.
16. Li, F.P., Cassady, J.R. and Jaffee, N.: Risk of Second Tumors in Survivors of Childhood Cancer. Cancer 35:1230–1235, 1975.
17. Hatfield, P.M. and Schulz, M.D.: Post-irradiation Sarcoma. Radiology 96:593–602, 1970.
18. Arseneau, J.C., et al.: Nonlymphomatous Malignant Tumors in Association with Intensive Therapy. N. Engl. J. Med. 287:1119–1122, 1972.
19. Coleman, C.N., et al.: Hematologic Neoplasia in Patients Treated for Hodgkin's Disease. N. Engl. J. Med. 297:1249–1252, 1977.
20. Toland, D.M., Coltman, C.A., Jr. and Moon, T.E.: Second Malignancies Complicating Hodgkin's Disease: The Southwest Oncology Group Experience. Cancer Clinical Trials, 1:27–33, 1978.
21. Smit, C.G.S. and Meyler, L.: Acute Leukemia after Treatment with Cytostatic Agents. Lancet 2:671–672, 1970.
22. Allan, W.S.A.: Acute Myeloid Leukemia after Treatment with Cytostatic Agents. Lancet 2:775, 1970.
23. Kaslow, R.A., Wisch, N. and Glass, J.L.: Acute Leukemia Following Cytotoxic Therapy. J.A.M.A. 219:75–76, 1972.
24. Greenspan, E.M. and Tung, B.G.: Acute Myeloblastic Leukemia after Cure of Ovarian Cancer. J.A.M.A. 230:418–423, 1974.
25. Reimer, R.R., et al.: Acute Leukemia after Alkylating-Agent Therapy of Ovarian Cancer. N. Engl. J. Med. 297:177–181, 1977.
26. Wall, R.L. and Clausen, K.P.: Carcinoma of the Urinary Bladder in Patients Receiving Cyclophosphamide. N. Engl. J. Med. 293:271–273, 1975.

THE
GOAL

20
THE GOAL

Although the highly sought "cure for cancer" does not exist, significant strides towards this goal have been taken along the proper path. The decade of the 1980s begins with more than 40% of all victims of cancer being cured of their disease. Previously fatal neoplasms, such as Hodgkin's disease, are now yielding in the majority of cases. Some tumors, like those of the vocal cords or testicular seminoma, are cured so frequently that recurrence is viewed with surprise. Surely, we have come a long way.

All cancers are not alike and it is naive to think that there ever will be *one* way to cure them. Rather, each type must be identified and separated from the others. Treatment must be appropriate to the needs of individual patients, not to abstract concepts.

Oncology in the future is as likely to be as different from that practiced today, as radiotherapy and chemotherapy are from the medicinal use of leeches. We must not be tied unalterably to the past, but, perhaps more importantly, we must not abandon unnecessarily the methods which already have proven beneficial, in the pursuit of something better. Progress can and usually must be made in small steps. Let us hope that we can learn from and thereby exploit the basic biology of tumors, so that we can select the most direct route to our goal.

INDEX

Page numbers in *italics* indicate figures; "t" indicates tabular matter.

Abdomen, irradiation of, reactions associated
    with, 216
Actinomycin-D, action of, 122–123, 134
  radiotherapy and, combined, 164
    decreased carcinogenic risk in, 253
    reactions associated with, 210
  reactions associated with, 210, 211, 213,
    216
Adenocarcinoma(s), cellular differentiation of,
    104–105
  of colon and rectum, 19–20
  of lungs, 16
  of prostate, relation of differentiation to
    biologic behavior of, 108
Adjuvant therapy, 101
Adriamycin, action of, 122–123
  and vitamin E, 137
  cardiac failure secondary to, 227
  in combination chemotherapy, 133
  in non-Hodgkin's lymphoma, 100
  radiotherapy and, 164
  reactions associated with, 211, 213, 216
Age, and sex, effect of, on likelihood of cancer
    occurrence, 183–188
  as factor in interpretation of success of
    therapy, 188
  effect of, on site of disease, 185
    upon clinical presentation of tumor, 186
    upon histologic type of tumor, 185–186
    upon prognosis, 188
    upon tumor management, 186–187
    upon tumor type, 183–185, 184t
Alimentation, artificial, in maintenance of nu-
    trition during cancer therapy, 201

Alkylating agents, in ovarian carcinoma,
    leukemia following, 252
Alopecia, chemotherapeutic agents causing,
    211
Alpha-fetoprotein, as marker, 50
Amenorrhea, chemotherapy-induced, 234–
    235
Aminopterin, congenital abnormalities related
    to, 239
Androgen therapy, in breast cancer, 112–113
Anemia, in cervical carcinoma, 159
Angiogram, *54*
  oxygenation of cancer cells and, 159
Apoptosis, definition of, 143
  examples of, 143–144
  in cancers, 144
Appetite, anti-cancer therapy decreasing, 200
Arteries, coronary, occlusion of, secondary to
    anti-cancer therapy, 227
L-Asparaginase, action of, 123
  acute reaction to, 208, 214
  in acute lymphocytic leukemia, 97
Astrocytoma, cellular differentiation of, 105
  grade I, 37
  grade IV, 37
Automobile exhaust fumes, as carcinogens,
    9–10

Basal cell carcinoma(s), cutaneous, 14
Biochemical abnormalities produced by
    tumors, 199–200
Biopsy(ies), blind, of bone marrow, 57
  confirmation of tumor, 47–48
  directed hepatic, 57

259